MY EPIDEMIC

An AIDS Memoir of One Man's Struggle
as Doctor, Patient and Survivor

Second Edition

Andrew M. Faulk, M.D.

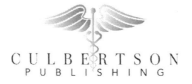

CULBERTSON
PUBLISHING

My Epidemic: An AIDS Memoir of One Man's Struggle as Doctor, Patient and Survivor. Second Edition.
Copyright ©2020 by Andrew M. Faulk. Previous edition copyright © 2019.
All rights reserved.

Cover art: TreeHouse Studios, Winston-Salem, North Carolina
Author photo: Lorinn Coburn

Poem "Memory Unsettled" by Thom Gunn is used with the permission of the Estate of Thom Gunn

Edited by Jerry Rosco.
Proofread by Daniel Stone and Shane Gildea.

Culbertson Publishing
info@culbertsonpublishing.com

ISBN Hardback 978-1-7334291-3-9
ISBN Paperback 978-1-7334291-4-6
Library of Congress Control Number: 2019913281

Printed in the United States of America

for my brothers

ACKNOWLEDGMENTS

In this endeavor a great many people gave of themselves. First of all I am indebted to Jerry Rosco, author of the biography *Glenway Wescott Personally* and editor of the Lambda Literary Award-winning journal *A Heaven of Words* and Glenway Wescott's *A Visit to Priapus and Other Stories*, who provided the comprehensive initial edit as well as patient direction and technical assistance throughout this undertaking. I want to express my deep appreciation for Anita Rachel Tierney, my good friend from my days at Columbia University, who took on the extraordinarily difficult task of transcribing the manuscript from its original handwritten form. Both Jerry and Anita contributed to my efforts through their heartfelt enthusiasm and unabashed partiality. Words fail me when I attempt to express my gratitude to Lorinn Coburn, who contributed remarkable clarity of thought and a profound understanding of life and relationships in ways I haven't always recognized. I am greatly indebted to Louis Bryan, Jr. and Shannon Biggs who generously gave me constructive criticism and invaluable suggestions, as well as Bob Coe, LCSW, who provided penetrating insights into the people and times of the Great Epidemic (now, unfortunately by necessity, renamed the AIDS pandemic). I am also tremendously grateful for Dick A. Bretto, Linda Gromko, M.D., Billy Tyler, Jr. and the late Bill Litts who contributed to my efforts through their unflagging inspiration and fervent certainty. The late Lynne Gaudinier-Bell was an extraordinary woman who is both much missed and fondly remembered. All of these people, in championing the project, reinforced my determination to complete what was a challenging re-examination of myself and history.

I am incredibly thankful for Thomas M. Reich, a man with striking abilities in wordplay and who has been a kind critic, an enthusiastic accomplice, a dazzling comedian and a constant friend. He has taught me that we cannot expect from others as much as we expect from ourselves, and he has given his best to this manuscript, and to me.

In particular I thank Mark Higgins, M.D. and Greg Pauxtis, M.D., my superb physicians, who, through the example of their own lives and work, taught me both the obvious and the extraordinary. I also want to acknowledge the invaluable support and contributions of Lawrence Otis Graham, Kurtis Opp, PA-C, Joseph Dunn, Teresa Gardiner, Nicola (Chris) Bucci and my cousin Gary Olsen and his remarkable wife Pat. I was also helped tremendously by proofreaders Dan Stone and Shane Gildea. I am profoundly indebted to John James Stevenson for so many things, that to review them all is impossible—he gave me the best of friendship and opened much of the world for me, including the wonders of Halley's Comet sailing over the ancient observatory of Chichén Itzá.

I wish to especially thank my late father, Ernest Faulk, for traversing what was a formidable distance in psyche and religion in order to mend a relationship and provide much inspiration and a quiet heart. My late mother, Wilma Faulk, contributed to this project in truly countless ways—from using a home chalkboard to tutor her reading-challenged 7-year-old son, to providing the magnificent example of graduating from college with honors, at the age of 48, and going on to teach other children in more formal settings. When my orientation was made clear, it was my mother who eventually came to the conclusion that the only thing my parents could do, finally, was love me. Which they proceeded to do without reservation.

No expression of gratitude would be complete, of course, without thanking my husband, Frank Jernigan, for providing constant support and occasional remark.

Besides all those named above, I also thank my patients, many described here, who gave me their trust and intimacy, insight and instruction, and much in the way of creating not only this manuscript but also the man I am today.

TABLE OF CONTENTS

MEMORY UNSETTLED

Your pain still hangs in air,
Sharp motes of it suspended;
The voice of your despair —
That also is not ended:

When near your death a friend
Asked you what he could do,
'Remember me,' you said.
We will remember you.

Once when you went to see
Another with a fever
In a like hospital bed,
With terrible hothouse cough
And terrible hothouse shiver
That soaked him and then dried him,
And you perceived that he
Had to be comforted,

You climbed in there beside him
And hugged him plain in view,
Though you were sick enough,
And had your own fears too.

—Thom Gunn

INTRODUCTION

This book is about my epidemic—a very personal experience with AIDS in which I found myself as doctor, patient, and survivor. Not only have I been infected with HIV for over 30 years, but I am a physician who limited my practice almost exclusively to those with HIV during one of the worst periods of the epidemic: 1984 to 1991. These were years in which the only thing medicine had to offer those of us who were infected, was the treatment of individual opportunistic infections and malignancies, and, as much as possible, a "good" death.

Being a physician with the same illness as that of one's patients can be profoundly disturbing. And AIDS was no ordinary disease: it was infectious and, from what we knew, always fatal. As time progressed, however, as the epidemic grew, so did a need for doctors specializing in, as much as was possible, this unknown disease. Medical personnel were needed who were willing to not only face the possibility of infection and death, but also treat the gay segment of the population which, although not particularly rare, was considerably distinct and not especially liked. A career in another area of medicine would have asked less of me, but our community was drowning in need. In becoming an AIDS physician, circumstances may have guided some of my steps, but the path was my own. Whatever treatment I knew, whatever insight I had, came from experience rather than books, the wards not the classroom. I realized that, in whatever capacity I could serve, I would. I knew where I belonged; my place was with my brothers.

In spite of my efforts to separate the two roles of doctor and patient, every patient's illness became a mirror of my own disease.

Every time I walked into an examination room I was seeing me, talking to me, diagnosing me—in every patient I saw, I saw myself. Throughout this period, exact statistics were unknown but I assumed I was part of the vast majority that would die relatively quickly; I had no idea that I would fall into an extraordinarily small group which appeared to live indefinitely. Of course my continuing to live defines me as a survivor.

It is my hope that this book will be a reminder of the role AIDS played in reducing the rampant homophobia with which we lived in the years before HIV. In 1987 homosexuality was illegal in half of US states and much of the world and, even as I write this, gay marriage is only legal in 28 countries. The diagnosis of AIDS forced many to come out as homosexual. With the onslaught of HIV, and the political and social organizations it began, a change in society's outlook came, for at last we were seen as what we had been all along: fathers and mothers, sons and daughters, brothers and sisters. Society's "discovery" of our ubiquitous presence, however, came at far too high a price—but it did come. And with this recognition came the enlightenment that our sexual orientation was of less consequence than our character (to paraphrase Martin Luther King, Jr.). This book records my perspective of the environment which played a significant part in changing our society from one of unapologetic homophobia to gradually expanding acceptance.

I was never a researcher, so this book is about serving patients "in the trenches" and the exhaustion and heartache which came from treating those with this extraordinarily lethal illness. I am haunted by my first four patients. I remember their names. I remember what they looked like. I remember them in greater detail than some friends I haven't seen for several years. After coming under my care, all four died within three months.

During the course of my practice, I participated in the care of approximately 50 patients who died, each as different as any person is from another. Some of their stories I've told here in order to document the pride and hope, sacrifice and courage, of those with HIV and their caregivers. In every patient I attempted to supplant fear and pain with ease and serenity. And for every person I helped face death, I helped prepare myself for the same.

I continued treating immunosuppressed patients until my own disease began to compromise my abilities. This book records how

I've subsequently carved out a life for myself which has been varied, full, and, for the most part, happy. I've lived my life largely in a sense of modified denial: I say "denial" because I live ignoring the consciousness I have a disease, "modified" for I take my medications religiously and consult my doctors with the same diligence. Others have documented this health crisis with tremendous empathy and eloquence, but I believe there are few physicians who have stood in my shoes and written about their experiences—few infected have written of treating those infected. This is the story of my epidemic: my personal and professional struggles with HIV and my orientation as well as my endeavors to provide my patients and friends with the best assistance possible in their walk off this planet.

* * *

Since the end of my practice, I've learned that the best method of dealing with loss is not the route of solitude and silence I usually chose. Occasionally in the following pages I explain that I lacked the time or energy to properly grieve—that my work demanded tunnel vision in order to be executed with efficiency and empathy. Such methods are and were unhealthy. It is impossible to run from, or attempt to postpone, emotions without experiencing significant consequences. It would have been better had I sought out supportive individuals or groups in which to process my turmoil and register my losses. But such insight was not in my emotional vocabulary at the time. It is now.

* * *

I must apologize to the great community of lesbians and straight allies who came to our aid in as varied, gritty and sacrificial ways as is possible. There's little mention of them here because my work didn't happen to overlap with their remarkable contributions. I can never express sufficient thanks, however, to this group of untiring people who gave of themselves from the very beginning of the epidemic.

* * *

Many will find the persistent use of masculine pronouns grating.

During the course of my career, by chance, I cared for only one woman with HIV and therefore the universal use of the masculine gives my notes an accuracy that what might appear to be a more even-handed presentation would not.

While I use literal descriptions for almost all of the people I write about, a few of my characters are composites of different individuals. In a spirit of respect and protection, names have occasionally been changed.

* * *

Most scientists believe that HIV originally came from a virus particular to chimpanzees in West Africa during the 1930s, and was eventually transmitted to humans through the transfer of blood through hunting. Scientists also believe that the first verified case of HIV is from a blood sample taken in 1959 from a man living in what is now Kinshasa in the Democratic Republic of Congo.

* * *

In terms of nomenclature, I have used "AIDS" and "HIV" interchangeably. H.I.V., human immunodeficiency virus, causes the disease AIDS, Acquired ImmunoDeficiency Syndrome. HIV primarily attacks the immune system. Not everyone with HIV has AIDS; AIDS is the late stage of HIV infection.

For ease in reading, when discussing the disease COVID-19, I have avoided using the name of the causative virus, SARS-CoV-2. Furthermore, in place of COVID-19, I have substituted "Covid-19" and "the coronavirus" to indicate both the disease and the virus. In point of fact, coronaviruses are a large family of viruses, but I have used "coronavirus" strictly in reference to the disease Covid-19. The number "19" in Covid-19 refers to the year of its appearance and naming: 2019.

The word "plague" is actually a very specific term in medicine referring to the bubonic, pneumonic and septicemic forms of the infections of the bacillus *Yersinia pestis*. In this book I have used "plague" in reference to HIV, Covid-19 and in the vernacular sense of general pestilence.

PART 1
PRACTICE

A HANDPRINT OF THE PAST

Well, this was the way it was. Or at least the way it was for me. For there is nothing in my story that makes it any more or less accurate than those told by so many others who lived through the worst days of the epidemic.

More than 30 years after I was told I was HIV-positive, I found myself with my husband, Frank, walking into a furnished house in Cazadero, California, to spend a weekend away from the routines of life. And there on the right side of the mantel was a "pinscreen," a curio consisting of a small lucite box of silver-colored metallic rods, a 3-D "executive" toy, maybe 10 by 8 inches, designed to capture the terrain of one's face, or hand, or whatever is pressed against it. If one flips the box over, however, all the metal rods fall back into their original, shapeless configuration. Like an old-fashioned Etch-a-Sketch, this toy could create an impression technically faithful, but easily wiped away.

It reminded me of visiting the apartment of my friend, Norman Nash, in the early 1990s, who showed me his own pinscreen. In his, poignantly, lay the handprint of his deceased lover. It held all the turmoil and sorrow of our time. Each time we visited his apartment in Elizabeth, New Jersey, he would survey it with a sadness and foreboding. The little device was never meant to capture a likeness permanently; its charm was in its transient preservation of an image which was easily erased by merely tipping it over. "I don't know what to do with this," he'd say. "I can never erase it, but I can't protect it forever."

JEFF
THE COMING STORM

During my years of medical school at the University of Washington, Seattle, in the early 1980s, I had a long-distance relationship with a New Yorker named Gene whom I met when I attended Columbia University. From time to time I would fly back to New York for this holiday or that and stay with Gene for a few days. It was during one of those visits that I learned of the death of a young handyman named Jeff. This was to be the first AIDS death of someone I knew. Jeff had been one of those relatively impoverished men in their late 20s/early 30s who hadn't been fortunate enough to attend college and weren't part of the class of excruciatingly handsome, gym-going, successful young professionals of the gay community. He was, nonetheless, clever, articulate, and incredibly resourceful in making a living in what could have been, for him, an overwhelmingly expensive and hostile Manhattan. He was in a group of men, wrestling without steady income, who were friends of Gene and his neighbor, Joseph, an artist in the same building.

Although we weren't close friends, Jeff and I knew each other, and occasionally heard about each other through Gene and Joseph. Gene and I had once visited Jeff's apartment and found him in the midst of writing a porn novel, not his first, an activity that supplied him some income. He also made the odd dollar installing home sound systems and producing small, battery-powered, light-emitting *objets d'art* which blinked and counted with colored lights.

Sometime during those years in the early 1980s I was visiting Gene and noticed Jeff's attractive little wall art—now with its blinking lights burnt out. At the time, Joseph was in the apartment on a small

ANDREW M. FAULK, M.D.

errand. Seeing the art silent and dark, I asked them about Jeff. He had suddenly fallen ill, Gene reported, and had entered the hospital and died within two weeks of some poorly-defined central nervous system disease. Numerous specialists had been called in on his case but to no avail. Once Jeff had passed away, as Gene had a key to Jeff's apartment, it had fallen on him to go with Jeff's father to unlock the door. In a scenario that was to be repeated over and over in those years, with different grieving family members in different homes, the two of them opened his apartment, and together worked through his various possessions. At some point they were both embarrassed to find sexual paraphernalia, and this inadvertent stumbling into the intimate details of Jeff's life made them feel horribly intrusive. As they went through the rest of his belongings, his tearful father repeated, "I don't know what to do with these things. I don't know what to do."

During my conversation with Joseph and Gene, Joseph was initially perplexed as he had confused Jeff with Scott, another one of his friends. Scott, unlike Jeff, had drifted away from him and the first evidence Joseph knew of a problem was when he had been out in Greenwich Village. Walking down Bleecker Street, Joseph had looked up to see Scott's apartment standing empty, for he had, in a similarly disturbing manner, died suddenly.

The three of us were thrown by the sudden death of the two men and the mysterious nature of their illnesses, but we realized later it had to have been AIDS. Our anxious astonishment was based on an earlier time when such youthful deaths were exceptional, before many of us began to exhibit the emotional shut-down of a population permanently stunned and bereft of the psychological energy required for grief. Bewildered, our review of these two early deaths was a pivotal moment for me—for all of us. The epidemic had already begun its terrifying machinations and, without fully understanding, we had begun to experience the sudden and incomprehensible loss of friends, acquaintances and neighbors.

In the beginning of medical school the long-distance relationship with Gene worked well: we saw each other at least twice a year. As our holiday reunions were infrequent, times spent together were all the more cherished. One semester I was even able to study in New York. I lived with Gene on the Upper West Side and the relationship didn't seem to miss a beat. Gene was my window on the artistic and literary world of Monroe Wheeler (a pivotal figure in New York's Museum of Modern Art) and the writer Glenway Wescott; Joseph became my view into the local social world. Through them I began to hear of the rising groundswell of AIDS deaths. Soon after Jeff had passed, I learned that the man to whom Jeff had once paid "key money" for a loft apartment, Larry Richardson, had died. Larry had been a Broadway stage designer and was in a crowd of prosperous New York men.

This group of more or less successful men, whom the rest of us greatly envied, was a segment of the population which seemed particularly blessed. Born with a baseline of good looks, gym workouts for these men seemed effortless and productive: they merely touched a weight and seemed to instantly hypertrophy. Following work, they exercised, came home, had a "power nap," and raced to the bars and bathhouses at the time when their more conventional peers were heading to bed. Out of the apartment at 11 or midnight, they socialized until two or three in the morning. And the next day they were up early doing household chores or getting to the gym before work. Their energy seemed boundless: they seemed to effortlessly juggle work, gym, social life, and the necessary daily chores of grocery shopping, bill paying, laundry, and cooking. Cleaning house was, perhaps, not performed as thoroughly as their gym workouts—not that there weren't plenty of obsessive-compulsive men whose apartments were so spotless that they more than compensated for the untidiness of some of their peers. The more worldly will also fault me for not taking into greater account those whose lives were routinely augmented by various pharmaceuticals. Besides this baseline of envy, most of my brothers lived under the abiding assumption that their better looking and more socially successful peers were having more sex, better sex than they. It is impossible to sort out how much of this was, in fact, real and how much was fantasy. But before AIDS the gay community was living in a continuation of 1960s' "free love" and promiscuity was valued not only for its inherent pleasure but also as a mark of freedom from the old strictures of a tyrannical society.

As Joseph's wider social circle mirrored that of the gay population as a whole, the escalating death toll was increasingly unnerving. At this point, the enormity of the number of deaths began to hit those like me who had wishfully assumed that only the most sexually promiscuous and drug-addled were at risk. After this assumption was proven wrong, our next misguided urban legend—which we wanted to believe—was that the epidemic was largely limited to the "players" among us: the political and social leaders, the most successful, the most handsome, those with the most resources to travel and those with the most contact with others. This assumption, too, was quickly proven wrong.

It soon became clear that anyone could die from AIDS—from the successful Wall Street executive to the "party boy" to the drug-ravaged homeless. If this terrible new disease could reach any of these, it could reach any of us.

THE PIED PIPER OF HAMELIN

In those days, the fairy tale of the Pied Piper of Hamelin was on my mind. It is a fable of an event which supposedly occurred in the 13th century involving a rat infestation of the medieval town of Hamelin, which ended successfully when a magical "pied piper" was employed to lead the rats away from town by playing his magic flute. After the task was completed, the story goes, the town fathers refused to pay him the agreed-upon sum. In retribution, the piper played his flute again, but this time the children of the village were the prey that followed the flautist into a magical opening in a rocky mountain from which they never returned. Now, in my tragic real-world rendering, there had to be a clear demarcation between those ahead and those behind. One can imagine a cut-off point at which those at the end of the line were saved. Was I at the head of the line— one who had enjoyed many sexual exploits and therefore would pay the highest price? Or was I at the end—one who had initially felt deprived and isolated, yet escaped the piper's song and lived to tell the tale? During the years that followed, my thoughts were to return to this analogy and this unknown again and again.

In the ensuing years I was to travel to New York many times, and each time the number of Gene and Joseph's acquaintances lost to mysterious illnesses rose at an accelerating pace. At this point, however, although the number of dead was increasing, no one with whom I was intimate had become ill. So the terror remained, for me, at abeyance. But this was to change all too soon.

In my third year of medical school at University Hospital in Seattle I saw my first AIDS case or, more accurately, witnessed its surroundings. Inside the hospital, a tented room had been constructed

ANDREW M. FAULK, M.D.

which used negative pressure isolation. This is a technique in which air pressure inside the room is kept below that outside of it so that when one enters, potential pathogens are swept inside; this prevents airborne diseases from escaping into the rest of the hospital. The partition of the room itself was such that, even in passing, one couldn't see the patient. I didn't participate in that unfortunate individual's care, I merely saw the attending physicians' moon suits from a distance. The hushed tones of the doctors involved and this extreme degree of isolation—as well as the fact that we students were not allowed any part of the case—spoke volumes. There always exists doctor-patient confidentiality which, of course, is taken very seriously, but in this case the usual clipboards and charting were hidden away and closely guarded. These were early times in the history of AIDS—the disease was a mystery and speculation ran wild about what caused this frightening destruction of the immune system and how it spread. While routes of infection were beginning to be determined, researchers weren't yet absolutely certain. In fact, the HIV antibody test hadn't yet been developed, but it was to come soon. For me, it was to come all too soon.

PROFESSIONAL SECRECY

In 1984 I graduated from medical school. I had had occasional visits to New York where I'd see Gene and my extraordinary friend from Columbia, Nita Tierney. At the UW I had important friendships with Linda Gromko, Ron Fletcher, and Connie Smith, but I didn't share the more intimate parts of my life with anyone at school. These were, on the whole, years of isolation—though not necessarily loneliness, as growing up gay in a homophobic world had accustomed me to, and prepared me for, solitude.

My policy then was simple: I would disclose my sexual orientation to no one until I had safely earned every degree that I wanted. I refused to be barred from obtaining any diploma, certificate or professional endeavor because I was gay. On a more fundamental level, I didn't want to have myself defined by others; I rejected being pigeon-holed into one overriding definition that would eclipse other parts of me. In service to this cause I also did not disclose to casual friends or acquaintances. If I hadn't had such a fixed policy, the judgments and decision-making would have been constant. It may have been anchored in paranoia, but it wasn't clear how any given institution would react to someone gay. My ambition was considerable. Would disclosure to the UW bureaucracy have resulted in termination? Even then, this was absurd. I was more fearful that homophobic individuals might quietly sabotage my career than any formal difficulty I might encounter.

Now, looking back from the safety and comfort of the second decade of the 21st century and distant from the Bible belts of America, my self-imposed isolation appears self-defeating and I review it with a certain amount of regret. But I shouldn't be too unforgiving with

ANDREW M. FAULK, M.D.

myself, for I grew up in a society considerably different than the one of today and it was precisely our epidemic that changed a world that younger people can scarcely imagine. Society has changed and I have grown wiser with age. If I had it to do over again, I believe I would be willing to chance sacrificing my professional career and reveal my orientation. But then I quite possibly would never have been able to help our community in the ways I did.

DR. LeFOU
CHILDREN'S ORTHOPEDIC HOSPITAL—
SCISSORS AND A FLASK

In my third year of medical school, I began a clerkship in pediatrics at the Children's Orthopedic Hospital of Seattle. If surgery was fueled by egotistic showmanship and hypertestosterone, then nurturing oxytocin-rich pediatrics was its opposite, at least according to conventional wisdom. But interestingly enough, my experience was not to be as warm and fuzzy as most medical students encounter. Our teaching attendant was a Dr. LeFou who thought of himself as something of a comedian. In the long white hospital jacket of an attending physician, he kept a pair of shears. It was his habit, I was to discover later, to suddenly produce these scissors and amputate the necktie of an unwitting student before the startled individual became aware of what was happening. He also believed that "Attending Rounds" with his students should be brief and, to guarantee such a routine, he offered to pay for students' breakfasts if rounds lasted less than 30 minutes. As this naturally truncated discussion, it ensured that instruction didn't take too much of his day.

The premature ending of our conversations had quite an effect on me and my trust in the system. When I mentioned my reservations about the built-in system ensuring brevity, it was one of my rare moments of confrontation and an impolitic impulse, to be sure. When we met for rounds a few days later, Dr. LeFou shocked me by brandishing his ever-present scissors and attacking my tie. The blitzkrieg by his pocketed scissors was his common *modus operandi* and what was left of my tie hung by some inglorious threads. In logical defense I suggested that my tie could have been, among other possibilities, a family heirloom. My criticism of his absurd maneuver made him all the more angry with me, for my comments on his teaching style were apparently already on his mind. For someone who so readily projected his horror of castration, my response was unforgivable. When the gravity of his reaction became clear, I made light of my resistance. But any sense of humor he may have had had vanished and he, an attending, felt disrespected by a lowly third-year medical student. He notified the school that my knowledge was inferior and my patient interaction suspect.

The administration immediately pulled me from the rotation: a report of a substandard doctor was not to be taken lightly. What followed was a month of sequestration and ancillary testing. My degree, my future profession, was in sudden doubt. And it had nothing to do with my sexual orientation but was based on my resistance to Dr. LeFou's castration anxieties!

It was a tough month for me. As did many of my peers from that particular period, I had suffered for years from the "Imposter Syndrome" of not fully believing that I deserved my position and so feared my "impostor" status would be exposed. Those four weeks, however, proved I was more than capable of my responsibilities. But after that anxious month I understood my position in the system was far more precarious than I had ever imagined.

Despite the restoration of my standing, I was appalled by the situation into which I had unknowingly stumbled. These were adults teaching adults—there should have been no room for the type of game-playing to which I had been subjected. Seeing the relationship between attending physician and student as something more transcendent than a game of cat and mouse, I had thought attendings were to provide instruction rather than have their psychological insecurities indulged. According to the Bible, "vengeance is mine, saith the Lord," but He would have no input into the slaying of this particular Philistine. In a juvenile act of revenge I am somewhat embarrassed to recount, I concocted my own retribution of fire and brimstone for Dr. LeFou. On random nights he would be awakened at 3 or 4 in the morning with a phone call for which he would, presumably, shake himself awake only to discover a disconnected phone. Should he have pursued the incidents, he would've found the calls couldn't be traced as they were placed from different UW hospitals and the phones involved were accessible to a great many hospital employees. It was regretful that he couldn't have known that this was punishment for a specific crime but, no matter, the child in me was gratified that Dr. LeFou was paying a price.

In my last year of medical school, I took the only elective course offered in virology. The specter of HIV was growing and I expected competition for one of the two available positions. But after registration I was surprised to find that I was the only one signed up for the rotation. Before the age of HIV, most sites for viral testing and research were in pediatric hospitals as it was commonly the pediatric population which fought serious viral infections. So it was with trepidation I once again walked the halls of Dr. LeFou's Children's Orthopedic Hospital. This time the experience couldn't have been more different: the work was largely research in a laboratory which had a relaxed, friendly atmosphere. The researchers had been working together for a long time and their relationships were based on shared work and shared success. The lab itself, made up of multiple booths with overhead safety fans separated by glass partitions, was astonishingly high-tech. As we worked we wore white paper throwaway suits, hats and shoe-coverings as well as clear plastic goggles. Toward the end of my six weeks, I was in the most central section of the lab when I heard a deep resonant chime of four notes. As I was in the middle of a task, I was only half-listening as a disturbingly calm woman's voice announced: "This laboratory has just sustained a biological accident. Please leave everything behind and walk to the nearest exit." The recording's content and delivery absolutely mesmerized me. The message was repeated. The glass doors had already begun to shush closed when I stirred myself out of this daze and scampered to the exit. One of our most capable researchers, an endearing and shy Iraqi ex-pat, had broken a flask; alone, she had remained behind as the glass doors closed. The other researchers and I looked at her forlornly as she, enveloped in the white uniform which covered her body, except for her goggled eyes, stared back at us with what I took to be calm acceptance before she methodically began the clean-up process.

The shattered flask had contained HIV-infected matter.

WITNESSING A NEAR-DEATH EXPERIENCE

During my senior year as resident at what was then the Pacific Presbyterian Medical Center of San Francisco (now California Pacific Medical Center, CPMC), an event occurred that was a direct contradiction of my personal beliefs—and perhaps an indication of a different kind of possibility. To be senior resident meant that I was supervising a junior resident and an intern who had the responsibility of admitting all patients that night who didn't require immediate intensive care. By definition this meant that I was responsible for admitting patients after 5 p.m. and running any "Codes" (emergencies) throughout the hospital, except those in the intensive care units.

Sometime in the early hours of the morning a Code was called. In this case, an older man's heart had stopped and he had ceased breathing. As he hadn't been in the hospital for a heart condition, he was without a cardiac monitor and the alarm had been somewhat delayed. It was my responsibility, as senior resident, to reach him as quickly as possible and orchestrate his revival.

From different places in the hospital, the respiratory team, the pharmacists, the nursing staff and I all rushed to his bed. When I reached the room the patient was unconscious and already receiving CPR as others were placing cardiac monitoring patches on his chest; a respiratory therapist was beginning intubation. He was a man somewhere in his early eighties who had been admitted to the medical floor that day. The nature of my duties was such that I never actually touched him, directing others to perform the manual operations such as chest compressions, intubation and starting a large-bore intravenous (IV) line. My duties were to direct the seven or eight others in the room while monitoring all the information available. It wasn't a particularly long intervention as a combination of electrocardioversion (electric shock to the heart), IV drugs and chest compressions revived his heart, although leaving him comatose. But the patient had survived and we congratulated ourselves on a successful Code. He was transferred to the Cardiac Intensive Care Unit (CICU) and I was left to my routine obligations of supervising the physical exams and admitting orders of the others on my team.

The next morning, as my admitting responsibilities were ending and another team took charge, a nurse in the CICU called me: "Dr. Faulk, you've got to come down here and see this for yourself—you must have run a hell of a Code!"

Sometime between 7:00 and 9:00 a.m. I found my way to the busy CICU and into this man's hospital bay. I was in my hospital scrubs as the previous night's work had left me disheveled and, as I had needed to discard my lab coat, I was without my name tag. There was no appreciable difference in my attire from all the other physicians, nurses and ancillary staff coming and going through his room that morning. As I parted the curtain of his bay, there was my patient sitting up in a chair and eating breakfast with his wife at his side.

Immediately upon seeing me, before I had spoken, he turned to her and said angrily, "That's the guy, that's the one who did it to me!" Above her remonstrations I asked him what it was I had done that so upset him. "You! You were the one who brought me back and you had no right!" He proceeded to tell me that he had been in a beautiful place—a place of tranquility, happiness and harmony with a benevolent world. He had been in the process of crawling into a green meadow through something like a wooden fence when, evidently with some violence, I had caught hold of him and dragged him back to the far different environment of his present surroundings. I went on to question him: how did he know I was the one who revived him? The night before, he had been wheeled out

ANDREW M. FAULK, M.D.

of his room comatose on a gurney. And, as I walked into his CICU bay, he had spoken before I had. He had neither seen me in the hours after the incident nor before my visit to his bay that morning. During the controlled chaos of the previous night, had he seen me from some place, above his bed perhaps?

No.

If he didn't know me by sight or voice, how could he know it was me? He didn't know how it was possible, but nevertheless he knew I was responsible.

Was he a religious man? Had he seen any personage such as Jesus?

No, neither. He had not been a religious man and, he insisted, this incident wouldn't change that. The only way this experience had affected him was that now he had no fear of death. He had been in a beautiful place, he told me, where he felt at one with a serene universe. Being a patient in an intensive care unit is bewildering, not only because of whatever ailments provoked the incarceration, but also for the constant intrusion of all manner of doctors, nurses and technicians, asking this or that while performing obnoxious examinations and distressing procedures. An intensive care unit, for those who aren't familiar with them, is a loud, busy, often unhappy place, where a patient receives many things, but neither seclusion nor serenity are among them.

I looked at him now with IVs, cardiac monitors, urethral catheter and nasal oxygen cannula, all producing a cacophony of disturbing beeps and buzzes. He looked up at me, simultaneously angry and forlorn—this was not where he had been—nor wanted to be. Throughout his denunciations his wife sat visibly disapproving of his remarks, especially those inveighing against me and my efforts. I was acutely aware of the perverse irony in the man's profound dissatisfaction with what I saw as a professional triumph. Nonetheless, he had been in a blissful place, and my "bringing him back" was reprehensible to him, and neither I nor any other doctor should ever do that to him again. The man asked me, how could he ensure that this calamity wasn't repeated?

I told him a simple "DNR" (Do Not Resuscitate) written on his chart by an on-site attending physician would mark his chart.

"Then do it," he said. "Do it right now!"

I walked out of his room and telephoned his attending. He

would be down soon from his regular hospital rounds, but if patient X was so determined to have an immediate change in status, he'd circumvent protocol and okay the DNR over the phone. I found the charge nurse, and she and he spoke. I firmly believe everyone should have ultimate control over their own body, especially when it comes to issues of life and death; I wrote the order and the patient's chart was flagged as DNR.

There was no easy, rational explanation for this incredible event. Was his vision of a transcendental world of peace and unity merely the result of signals from a disrupted, dying brain—as studies consistently reproduce? Was his identification of me an indication of a presently-unknown means of communication? I can believe that science has not yet discovered all the ways in which we converse: it is not beyond the pale for other, presently unknown, forms of information transference to exist. Nevertheless we have no scientific confirmation of such phenomena. But even with some undiscovered form of human communication, to an outside "civilian," a Code is a chaotic affair; a routine Code, as was this one, would test the limits of any such aptitude. With the various nursing, respiratory and pharmacy personnel reporting the state of their various tasks and the patient's response, the room can become a baffling uproar of activity. Someone unfamiliar with this emergency event—or unconscious—could easily be perplexed not only by who was doing what, but also who was in charge. How would communication in these circumstances translate into an ability to connect my "transmission" with the physical me? And how could a brain suffering from oxygen deprivation activating the neural signals of death be able to identify my particular "voice"?

I have always been impressed by the education I received at the University of Washington School of Medicine. There it was taken for granted that an unconscious person had the ability to hear and, on some level, understand. My irascible gentleman may have heard elements of the commotion, but to identify the individual with ultimate responsibility was a stretch. Besides, the next morning when I walked into his hospital room, he had recognized me before I had spoken or could be identified by scrub color, name tag or activity.

Once immersed in HIV care, I tried to will myself to believe in a greater cosmic structure than what I could perceive. I wished for a universe, a god (however ill-defined), that would take my

ANDREW M. FAULK, M.D.

dying patients into a heaven of some kind. Into some comforting afterlife—be it Christian, Muslim, Hindu, Shinto, or whatever—some serene existence without pain, sorrow or isolation. Yet in spite of motivation and this compelling involvement in a near-death experience, I can't will myself to believe in heaven. Perhaps one day I'll find it possible to believe—to choose to believe—in a higher power without the nagging sensation I am deceiving myself. Until then this episode, whether due to science or the supernatural, remains the most powerful cognitive dissonance of my life.

OUR CONTRACT WITH SOCIETY

Before the 1983-1984 definitive conclusions about routes of infection, HIV had a paralyzing effect on the medical system and sometimes a form of anarchy emerged. In the earliest years, I witnessed food trays abandoned by the food and kitchen staff outside the door of HIV patients, relatives too frightened to walk into their loved ones' rooms and funeral homes rejecting the deceased for mortuary preparation and burial. By the time I moved to Los Angeles in the late 1980s, however, such incidences had ended altogether.

I feel solidarity and great pride with those physicians who dealt with plagues throughout history. These overwhelming times (the 1980s and early 1990s) revealed the best in my colleagues. In the earliest years, when so little was known about AIDS, I only once saw any type of medical personnel express the slightest hesitancy in treating an AIDS patient. Although I admit I did hear of some physicians refusing to care for HIV patients, the exception that proved the rule was when I witnessed a doctor turn down a patient who was bleeding. Dr. X in the E.R. remonstrated that she had children and that the risk was too great. On the whole, however, there was no task beneath their status: our physicians, whether in training or attending, would pick up a food tray on the floor left outside a patient's room and then matter-of-factly deliver it. In addition, I saw more than one physician volunteer to staff shifts and care for certain bleeding patients when there were possible risks of HIV infection. An early AIDS researcher, Dr. Paul Volberding, dealt with recurring nightmares that he had become infected by patients and spread the disease to his children. I have never been more proud of my fellow physicians as when, without self-consciousness

ANDREW M. FAULK, M.D.

or pause, complaint or question, they would perform hundreds of examinations and procedures which sometimes presented risks of infection—but almost all requiring the simple act of touch.

I am proud to add that the nurses involved in treating those with HIV were of such constitution that the exposures they encountered did not intimidate them in the slightest. They were without trepidation in their devotion to their charges. Although they may have flinched from time to time when splashed or sprayed with blood or other bodily fluids—as we all did—their speed and thoroughness in their duties bespoke a fearless dedication to the wellbeing of these patients.

Throughout my career I always instructed the nurses and others caring for my patients that, if they debated calling me at all, they should just call. If a medical problem unexpectedly turned into a more difficult situation, hesitating to call me would only have made the situation worse. There was always a chance an assessment could indicate nothing amiss, but I believed that when I "signed up" to be a physician, I wasn't just accepting the title but the responsibility as well. I was committed to patient care even when, later, it began to affect my own health. It was with this understanding that I encouraged the nurses working with me to show no reticence about calling me no matter the hour. I swore to them that they would never be criticized for that 3:00 a.m. call.

To be a physician meant that one had signed up for both the good and the bad. To me this was the agreement, our contract with society.

A MENACE PRESENT

The post-graduate training system had matched me in Internal Medicine with CPMC in San Francisco. Internship I knew would be ghastly, with unbelievable hours of work. What I couldn't know was the personal upheaval that was to come.

That year of internship was one of the hardest of my life. Because of the fantastic hours of work—I once clocked 110 hours of work in one week—there was little time for friends, but nevertheless I had a few. I had met Louis Bryan during my interviews in San Francisco and he became a good friend. I still had Gene Spencer, although he was a continent away. I managed to meet Dick Bretto that first year—a generous, practical man who remains a close friend to this day. But those kinds of hours didn't make for much of a social life and the other interns, the attending physicians, and the nurses soon became nearly my entire social world.

Early in that year it fell to me to do the "History and Physical" of an AIDS patient with *Cryptosporidium*, an organism which produces, among other things, life-threatening watery diarrhea. It was known that cryptosporidiosis patients in San Francisco, mysteriously unlike other locales, died quickly after diagnosis, therefore I knew that our patient was not long for this world. It was up to me, I felt, to make his illness, his life, count. In an environment in which the science was so unknown, I took this opportunity to get as complete a medical, social, sexual and recreational drug use history as possible. I was still living in a world in which we all wanted to believe that anything this terrible had to have a susceptibility brought on by the patient himself. (The term "victim" is disempowering and grates on my sensibilities.) Surely it was some treacherous combination of drugs in concert with wild promiscuity—far outside of my harmless cannabis and the infrequent sex that I thought left me safe. I quizzed this man as thoroughly as possible. To his credit he answered every one of my questions in explicit detail. It became obvious that he felt the extraordinary importance, the overriding urgency, of what he and I were doing and he wanted to help in the fight. What exposure might he have had at work? In his home? Was he breathing fungus, pollution or bacteria? Any unresolved systemic disease or infection? Had his sexual contacts been diagnosed with an immunosuppressive disease? Diseases in his family? Malignancies, infections, immunosuppression or hyperimmune conditions?

Perhaps the attending physician sensed my fevered search for complexities or co-factors which would make the patient stand out from the crowd of other gay men who were apparently left untouched. My notes were too extensive for him to be a routine patient of any type, even for a patient with AIDS. After reading my meticulous work-up approvingly, the attending doctor's only comment was to ask whether or not I was planning a career in research.

The patient would be dead soon and his story would have to be told through our records. Perhaps in them, and in the thousands of other histories from the thousands of other patients, could be found a clue leading to the extermination of the virus. My hope was that my pages of notes would speak for him after his death and that his sacrifice wouldn't have been in vain. It was clear that he, too, understood the profound importance of our work and, in that hospital room that day, he wasn't only a patient—he was a vital collaborator.

THE WORLD TURNED UPSIDE DOWN

In the Fall of 1985, there were several days in which I found notes attached to my front door from a group wanting to interview me for a study. Cryptically, there was no information on its focus, who was conducting it or why I had been chosen. When at last they knocked on my door when I was at home, I discovered they were from the US Centers for Disease Control (CDC) and were studying AIDS. Would I take part in their study? Absolutely! I would do whatever I could to help hunt down this assassin. But why my door, why me? Later I was to discover that choosing subjects entirely at random is one of the best techniques for optimum statistical accuracy. I made an appointment for their clinic and was soon answering an exhaustive questionnaire that included my sexual history and recreational drug use and my blood was drawn at a nondescript site near what was then Children's Hospital. When my part in the study began, there was no test for the virus—but that was soon to change.

I can no longer remember how many times I was to answer questions and have my blood drawn during the months which followed. But it was on October 2, 1985, that the researchers asked me if I wanted to know the results of the newly-developed HIV antibody test. Although I didn't realize it, I was completely unprepared for my results. I didn't think about—hadn't thought about—the repercussions of an answer in the positive. My nonchalance was testament to my certainty that I had had less sex than my peers and I was therefore negative; I was certain that I was at the end of the Pied Piper's bewitched queue, not the beginning. Such was my denial.

The test was positive for HIV antibodies: I was infected.

I had been near enough to the front of the Hamelin-piper's

line after all—the terrible mountain had closed behind me, not in front. Nothing in my life would ever be the same. I know no word that would be hyperbole in describing that terrible moment of understanding. To mention the sudden dizziness or the sensation of blood instantly draining from my face would be to trivialize my reaction. Clinical experience wasn't necessary to know that I had been given a death sentence. I harbored no illusion that I was to survive this disease; I was as mortal as my brothers and just as there was no magic bullet for them, there was none for me. Had I received the diagnosis of any number of cancers, I believed, I would have had a more certain future: my prognosis would have had wiggle room. But that was not the case. On that October afternoon in 1985, my life was changed forever.

The researchers were well prepared. Would I like to talk with a psychologist? I felt so knowledgeable in medicine that I believed such a meeting would end up being like me talking to myself. What would a psychologist know that I, in the opposite position, would not? What could they say that I wouldn't say to a patient in a similar situation? That day I misjudged the value of what therapists have to offer. Although they couldn't have changed my status, they could have started me on the way to acceptance and developing the emotional tools I would need for the rest of my life.

Upon walking out of the clinic, I spent an hour hunting for my car. I had parked directly in front of the clinic and now its location was a mystery. At the age of 30, I had been diagnosed with a lethal illness. I was certain my career was ended, that my relationships were finished and my life was over. National Public Radio was playing on the car radio as I drove away from the clinic; it was reporting the death of Rock Hudson, the first major celebrity to die from AIDS.

I am not sure how I managed to remain a competent physician during those first few weeks after I learned my status, but I carried the information alone, telling no one. What I, the physician, would have told me, the patient, would have been to say yes to psychological counseling, for such a burden was too much for any person to bear alone.

But for years I didn't tell anyone—I didn't see a mental health professional. And for years I persisted in the same mistake I made that afternoon. I kept this inside. I told no one. For years after I left medicine, I mistakenly assumed that if I couldn't give answers, I had nothing to say—that the telling of my story was only valid if it could calm horror, manage sorrow or allay physical pain. Now I realize what many people have understood: our individual histories are rich in solace and hope, that in telling them, and listening to them, we exercise our humanity and that they frequently give healing where medications and treatment cannot. Now I realize that simple words strung together have the ability to provide relief where there is no remedy. That is my hope with this story of the epidemic—that it may be useful for physicians and patients in some other ordeal of plague.

I agonized over whether to end my career in medicine. Even though I had struggled for so many years, it hadn't yet truly begun. In order to become a physician, I had calculated an academic trajectory years in advance. I was particularly drawn to Stanford because of its West Coast location and proximity to San Francisco—a city famous for its gay community and natural beauty. I had applied there every year since 1974, first for undergraduate college, then as a transfer student in my sophomore year, then for medical school, then for an internship program, and finally for an Internal Medicine residency. I was turned down—again and again. In fact, I was to receive a rejection letter from Stanford the year after my last application— apparently my name was in their admissions computers with some permanence. I could paper a small bathroom with their rejections.

Since 1975, I'd chosen college courses to facilitate entry into medical school, taking classes in the summer with weekends full of homework and concentration. Judging universities against each other is a fool's errand, but I had transferred from Georgetown to Columbia in a perception that Columbia would be a better launching pad for a medical career. Despite constructing my strategies so carefully, all my planning, my years of education and training and the years of work and sacrifice were no defense against the damage that this virus could do.

Outside of work I did nothing for two weeks as I wrestled with the impossibility of my situation. The next one and a half years of training, should I live that long, would be filled with uninterrupted stress and crushing exhaustion destructive to my immune system. Maybe I had only months to live—was this how I wanted to spend my last days? Clearly continuing my residency would shorten my life. While I knew and respected those who live to work, I was about to discover whether that was my truth as well. At the end of those

ANDREW M. FAULK, M.D.

two weeks of contemplating my future, I scheduled an appointment with Dr. John Gamble, the Chief of Medicine of CPMC, in order to resign my position. It was time for me to stop living in the future and begin living in the present.

In those dark years of the 1980s, there was public debate concerning the safety of HIV-infected physicians treating HIV-negative patients. Although routes of transmission had been determined in 1983, the information took time to seep into public consciousness and society's anxiety continued for several years. Confronted with such a little-known and terrifying disease which had no truly effective treatment, politics and ignorance spread disinformation and fear. Already nervous about becoming infected, those uneducated, or disbelieving, about the route of HIV transmission were worried that HIV-positive doctors might infect their patients. In spite of the science, this persistent apprehension spilled over into politics and the legal world. Could patients become infected with HIV through infected physicians? Should infected doctors be prohibited from practicing? In 1985 California Rep. William Dannemeyer introduced a bill in Congress to prohibit anyone with AIDS from working in the healthcare industry. Long before President Clinton's military policy, it became a "don't ask, don't tell" era for HIV-positive physicians.

It is difficult to describe my feelings that day. Even in Dr. Gamble's office I was to remain essentially alone—I couldn't tell him that I was HIV-positive because of the possible legal ramifications concerning the patients I had already treated. This was unknown legal territory. Had I disclosed my HIV status to Dr. Gamble, the gears of the legal system would have likely engaged. My HIV status could have opened the hospital to liability even though we knew that transmission was limited to exchange of body fluids.

So instead I told Dr. Gamble that the hours were unmanageable and the stress overwhelming. I was resigning my position.

Dr. Gamble listened thoughtfully to my resignation and, instead of accepting it at face value, replied that he didn't want the program to lose me. I was one of their best interns, he responded, and he was considering the program's loss even more than my own.

"What, Dr. Faulk, do you need?"

I was incredulous—what did I need? Throughout my academic years in medicine, the ratio of applicants to positions was always so high that we knew we were easily expendable. Should we be unable or unwilling to perform as required, there were others who would be only too happy to replace us. But having carefully weighed my health against my residency, I wasn't prepared to consider half-measures. I told Dr. Gamble that I would need a month off. I was absolutely certain my request would be refused.

"What else do you need?" he quietly responded.

In all my planning I hadn't anticipated flexibility. I was astonished. What else?

The option to take another month off whenever I needed it, I said. Gamble was relentless. "And what else?" After taking a month off now and retaining the option to do so again at any time, if I could end stress whenever I wanted, perhaps I could continue my career! I could think of nothing else I needed.

His wisdom was strikingly apparent in his last question: would I be able to finish out the day? A doctor identified as troubled to a hospital administrator was not to be taken lightly. Although stunned by what had just occurred, I said yes, of course I could finish out the day.

I started that month by lying in bed for two weeks watching TV and drinking beer—a curious choice as I am not much of a drinker and I don't like beer. In retrospect, I should have sought counseling, but I struggled on my own—without help or audience. I didn't even venture out to gay bars where, even keeping my secret to myself, I could have had some support. Aside from re-thinking my career, I needed to generate a new self-image: a person with a terminal illness who could enjoy whatever life he had left.

In the ensuing years when I was to deliver an HIV test result to others, I would tell my devastated patients not to give up hope and, that in every epidemic throughout history, there were a number of survivors. Although I was always to encourage this optimism, the percentage of those who did well appeared to be incredibly small and, knowing this, I never assumed such a possibility for myself. The exact numbers may have been unknown but preliminary anecdotal reports were grim. I had no expectation of survival. Over the years I've contemplated again and again what my behavior would have been had I not been infected. Picturing such a state, I've always imagined that I would have locked myself in my career and in my apartment even more tightly than I had.

BILL OWEN, M.D.
FINDING A PHYSICIAN FOR MYSELF

After the roller coaster descent of learning that I was HIV-positive, I had to refocus my energies and, for the first time in my life, find a physician for myself. Doctors were advertised, occasionally with photos, in *Frontiers* (the local gay "rag"). Before contacting anyone I investigated a prospective physician's hospital affiliation—I couldn't end up being admitted to my own hospital or one closely affiliated. I found one of the doctors known for excellent HIV care, Dr. Bill Owen, who was associated with another hospital network. There was a considerable wait to see him, but I would white-knuckle the delay for the benefit of being cared for by someone well-versed in HIV.

He was thorough and knowledgeable in a way that assured me that when things began looking bad, he would perform well—hopefully with brilliance. One of the advantages of being on the inside in the world of medicine is the sense of connectedness one feels with other doctors and staff and the lack of surprise with whatever medical strategy may follow. After that first examination it was time to get my labs drawn. I sat in a hard plastic chair at the end of a long, green linoleum corridor which smelled of disinfectant and dread. How sick was I? My new doctor told me to wait for the lab results to return before I went home.

After 20 minutes, he walked out and informed me that he needed to re-check the platelet count. The tests showed thrombocytopenia (low platelets), which could be an early indication of HIV progression and a serious problem. Or it could be due to a simple and common lab problem. As I began examining myself for bruises, which would indicate inappropriate bleeding, another blood sample was taken. I sat in that hallway for another 20 minutes of waiting and then the answer came back: no, it was just a frequent lab hiccup. For the first time I was seeing the nightmare that chronic medical care would entail, the first feeling that it could well be unbearable, that it could all be simply too much. It would've been good at that moment, or at least better, if I hadn't been sitting there alone. The majority of my past relationships had ended poorly, but at this moment it would've been so much better to have had another person present. I internally debated my situation; I was okay, I told myself. Well, no, it was terrifying, but there were, after all, painkillers and anti-anxiety drugs, mind-numbing by either one route or another. Being a physician I could stay in the loop—as much as I wanted to be in the loop. But to be faced with the end of my career, after I had gotten so far; surely the world must be playing a cruel joke on me. Often in training I had felt like an adolescent because I was always in school without an income or days off. But now, here I was, stepping off the planet before I'd had the chance to live like an adult in an adult's world.

On my second or third appointment with Dr. Owen, a writer who was doing an article on Dr. Owen and AIDS wanted a photo of him examining a patient. Would I be willing to be that patient? I was initially unwilling, but thought better of it and allowed them to take a photo when they agreed to only show my back with Dr. Owen facing the camera. I refused to be photographed for I was feeling some embarrassment about having the disease—not only for the route of infection. I've discovered that there is some amount of shame, it seems, with any disease: if one can feel it with a non-infectious "innocent" illness such as multiple sclerosis, then it certainly is felt in HIV. I am not immune to such feelings, so I am glad I never saw the photo.

The Christmas break of 1985 was the most emotionally turbulent school break I have ever had. As if to emphasize the mind-bending horror of HIV infection, through a mutual friend in Seattle I learned that a gay physician I knew there had developed AIDS, began living in a tent in his backyard and died after three months. This of course was nothing compared to the news that I was HIV-positive. But I was in for greater sorrow and upheaval: I was to lose my major source of emotional support. That year I flew to Los Angeles as Gene had changed jobs and moved there; he, too, had been tested and was, thankfully, HIV-negative.

I hadn't noticed it before, perhaps it hadn't been there before, but Gene was now using a sing-song voice to announce the illness or death of anyone with AIDS whether they be friends, acquaintances or celebrities. It was the same tone a mother might use to say to a child, "I told you not to do that, and you did it anyway." While it is difficult to describe spoken tone on paper, I have no trouble describing how it made me feel—I was alone when it came to my status. It was a stance, communicated sideways, that said those with HIV were responsible for their illness. As I was HIV-positive, his reaction to my status created a separation; before, I was part of an "us," now I became part of "them." Gene was disconnected from those of us with HIV, and over time it became more and more painful. Even though we had a long history, and I loved him dearly, I ended the relationship just the same.

AIDS, sadly, unraveled some of our community's fabric as well. For even in the gay community, among a few here and there as in Gene's case, I had come to detect occasional subtle, and not so subtle, messages which signaled a psychological distancing between those with and those without HIV. Early on there was much fear and finger-pointing in our community by those reaching for the false sense of security that came from believing AIDS was caused by the use of recreational drugs—principally "poppers" (butyl- and amyl-nitrite). Although they eventually dropped off, early on in my practice I heard a great variety of conspiracy theories, such as a belief that the US Government developed and was spreading AIDS as a method of eradicating homosexuals.

On occasion I felt condemned for my HIV status—condemned along with my brothers—for an assumed promiscuity which those who were HIV-negative now disowned. HIV represented sexual activity itself and occasionally it seemed that as I had, presumably, enjoyed sex without restriction, some pay-back, some retribution, was in order. At times when I felt judged by gay men, I sensed an element of unspoken envy. The message that we with HIV were deserving of our disease was an echo of the one broadcast by that slice of the heterosexual community that was homophobic and unaffected by the epidemic and comfortable with any reason to condemn us.

Obviously, all of this failed to take into account that all that is required for infection was one exposure to one person.

Like pregnancy.

A DIFFERENT WAY OF LIVING

I now found myself with a very different *Weltansicht* from the young. Not only was I not indestructible, I could be close to dying without objective signs. Any bump or discoloration of the skin could be nascent Kaposi's Sarcoma. Any cough or tickle in the chest could be budding PCP. Any headache or simple act of forgetting could be evolving AIDS dementia or PML (progressive multifocal leukoencephalopathy, a viral infection of the brain). After my initial visit with Dr. Owen and the scare of thrombocytopenia, my T-cells were found to be in the high 300s.[1] (At the time, as in so much else, we had no test for viral burden—another test helpful in determining extent of infection and/or timing of approaching illness.) This was significant as most HIV-related diseases appeared to be occurring below a threshold of 200 T-cells and, if below 100, death was usually imminent. But as I was to emphasize with my patients, we simply didn't know the exact correlation between disease and T-cell count in any one individual. Although the long-term survival rate appeared to me to be—in a non-scientific, anecdotal guess—10%, this survival rate didn't apply to those with T-cell counts lower than 200. But even the information concerning T-cell counts wasn't established conclusively: there was the question about the status of T-cell function. Was it possible someone's T-cells might be more effective, or less effective, than usual? Perhaps this explained such cases as the man I treated who lived nearly six months with T-cells below 50 (he joked that there were so few he named them). Nothing could be absolutely certain: we were, after all, creatures of biology.

It was about this time that I developed a small, flaky, psoriasis-like patch beneath my left eye. It was somewhat itchy but without other identifying features. From the beginning of the epidemic, most patients with full-blown AIDS had a pronounced seborrheic dermatitis—a red, flaking rash, worse in and between the eyebrows, above and on the sides of the nose, bridge of the nose and on the chin. My solitary site, about the size of a nickel, was unusual for HIV in its location and clearly-defined borders, but I gave it a weight that it didn't deserve. For me it only confirmed what my lab tests showed—I was HIV-positive and my immune system was possibly damaged. Noticing this small lesion, as minor as it was, colored my perceptions and threw the dark, unexamined, edges of my life into sharp relief. How often had I been dishonest or unkind? How frequently was I judgmental or impatient? The disease reached into my consciousness and made me review my values and integrity.

Maybe my preoccupation would have been lessened by sharing my fear with others. However, I knew confiding in others in the medical community, as educated as they were, was tricky for it could have possibly jeopardized my career. I didn't feel I had the energy or resources to be a legal test-case for employing HIV-positive physicians. Thoughts of being questioned about my HIV status brought back memories of being asked earlier in my life if I were gay—those answers shame me to this day. It was an abhorrent throw-back in time that once again, should they arise, I might need to finesse such questions. It was an uncomfortable paradox of my time and situation that my equanimity was found in neither admitting nor denying my status. It was a solitary road.

Besides dealing with my own fears of HIV acceleration, there was another reason for feeling alone. Besides the burden of facing a decline in my personal health, there was a heaviness in terms of societal acceptance and support. These were dark times for gay people and I felt the weight; the early 1980s saw a toxic mix of fear of the virus and increased homophobia. It was inevitable that the disease would sooner or later be linked to us as if we were the cause and that the distinction between being gay and having AIDS would become blurred. To the homophobic, or insulated, the distinction between homosexuality and AIDS could be difficult to grasp; not all gay people had HIV, not all HIV-infected people were gay. Didn't it make sense to just assume that a Venn diagram overlap was complete—that all gay people had AIDS? And distancing oneself from gay people could bring protection from AIDS? Although my

HIV status was, obviously, not publicized, there were moments when I felt like an uninvited leper at society's table.

At the same time we were dealing with the parallel issue of the "forced outing" of gay people which often came with their AIDS diagnosis. I was present at bedside on several occasions when my patients were subjected to cruel rejection by their families as they simultaneously learned of their son's diagnosis and his sexual orientation. While I couldn't appreciate it at the time, these solitary incidents, as excruciating as they were, eventually contributed to a huge advancement in the acceptance of gay people and our movement for full legal rights and social acceptance. In a binary world of "us" and "them," for mainstream Americans we were "them." But the epidemic served an unexpected purpose: yes, we were "them," we were gay, but to the surprise of society, and even a few of us, the epidemic showed we were everywhere. And once everyone discovered our identities, even though it may have been only one individual at a time, discrimination was on the path to extinction.

Few people are willing to take away the job or apartment of their gay son or grandson.

ROBERT HAUSER, M.D.
PERCOCETS AND A GUN

I'll never know if the gun was loaded that day. To the onlooker it may have appeared to be bravery, but I was responding less as someone with bravery and more as someone already facing a death sentence.

As residents and interns, twice a week we would hold clinics during which we would treat those living in the neighborhood. In my last year of residency, 1986-1987, I was supervising a psychiatry intern in our clinic. Occasionally interns heading for psychiatry feel a little less capable in the "hard" science of high octane medicine, but an internship in medicine is necessary in order to be licensed. Robert Hauser was gay and as insecure and weighted down as any of our psychiatry interns. He was terrified at being thrown into the enormous pool of technology. Whenever I was on-call with him, I did my best to boost his confidence while paying a little extra attention to his work. On more than one occasion I had reassured him that he would do well. And when he expressed those moments of panic and futility, my message was consistent—he would get through this without problems and survive internship hell. I was Robert's cheerleader.

It was during one of these clinics that I heard a slight scuffle in the outside hall and looked up from my notes to see one of the nurses who worked in the clinic, and whom I knew well, rush into the conference room. "Dr. Faulk," she said, "we need you in the hall right away!" I was expecting an unconscious cardiac patient on the floor—what I found surprised me.

There in the hallway stood my insecure intern, Robert, standing stiffly and looking me right in the eye with a steely calmness I will

ANDREW M. FAULK, M.D.

always remember and admire. Standing behind him, slightly to the side, stood a man with dark, greasy hair in his early thirties. In his right hand he held a gun pointed at Robert's back. I've never been a hunter and I'm not used to seeing guns—their appearance unsettles me. Standing 25 feet away, my eyes traveled from the gigantic gun to Robert's eyes to the disheveled man and back to the gun.

As I entered the hall, the man with the gun was talking. "Why won't you give me Percocets? I need them and you know it!" The nurse to whom he was talking stood motionless and looked at me. Another nurse, in the distance behind, was at her grey metal desk frantically dialing for security.

I said the only thing I could think of: "Oh, Sir, we don't allow guns in the hospital—they frighten the patients." He said he didn't care, we were going to listen to him.

We did.

"I'm hurtin' and those sons-a-bitches aren't doing nothin' about it!"

My mind was racing. I had HIV; my fate was already sealed. I hoped that death from a gunshot wound would be quick. As I began walking to him I said, "You know, Dr. Hauser doesn't control pain management. I do. If you're going to point that thing at anyone, it should be me." I swallowed hard as he adjusted his aim and trained the pistol on my belly. Robert didn't move. As I reached the man I said, "You don't want to hurt anybody," and grasped the barrel, motivated in that moment by the thought that if he fired, I hoped my death would be quick… and painless. I was shocked; he allowed me to take the gun out of his hand. Security arrived, the drama ended and Robert Hauser had survived another day, a day infinitely more demanding than most.

I had been more at peace facing a potentially fatal gunshot wound than the possibility of a prolonged AIDS death.

TOMMY GORDON
MY YOUNGEST LOSS

I had rotations in the Intensive Care Unit (ICU) of CPMC as an intern and resident on and off during the years 1984 through 1987. It was during my internship year there that I cared for the youngest AIDS patient I ever saw. Perhaps the memories have acquired a more emotional patina than the events at the time, but I doubt it. In my early years as a physician, many AIDS patients ended up on ventilators—usually as a result of *Pneumocystis jirovecii* pneumonia which, at that time, we knew as *Pneumocystis carinii* pneumonia and called PCP for short. (In order to avoid confusion, "PCP" is still used.) I was too inexperienced, too untrained, to have firm opinions on whether those thought unlikely to recover should be placed on ventilators.

Tommy Gordon was one of our earliest AIDS patients. He was particularly memorable because he was admitted to the ICU at age 17; his 18th birthday occurred there while he was on a ventilator (a machine that mimics natural breathing and so infuses the lungs with oxygen). I had not admitted him to the hospital, or the ICU for that matter, and during the entire time I cared for him I never exchanged one word with him as he was unconscious. There wasn't even a moment of meaningful eye contact, as he was heavily sedated and his eyes were taped shut to save his corneas from the damage of infrequent blinking. In the bed he looked small, thin and pale. He may have had visitors but I don't remember any. I heard from his admitting medical team that when he was questioned about how many men he had had sex with, he responded with, "How many days are there in a year?" He was open about his trade; he was a hustler.

So there we were with a teenager on a ventilator. I wasn't alone when I debated with the ICU attending physicians whether or not his ventilator should be discontinued and the natural course of the disease be allowed to end his suffering. We doctors in training, to the person, argued that he should be allowed to die. His family, who lived somewhere in the San Joaquin Valley, were not involved in his care, but with much difficulty his mother had been contacted. She had said that her home duties—a job and a child—didn't permit her to visit and she abdicated any responsibility for his care to the hospital's attending physicians. In spite of our clear and persistent explanations of his terminal diagnosis, the mother's response revealed a blasé attitude and disturbing denial. "You do what you think is best. Tell Tommy hello and I hope he gets better fast."

The Intensive Care attending physicians, thus given ultimate license, ruled that his life support be continued. They argued, "What if you allow him to die and a cure for AIDS is discovered tomorrow? It's unlikely but possible. How would your decision stand then?"

Tommy Gordon died on the next to the last day of my first Intensive Care rotation. With the ICU team I had cared for him the entire six weeks, during which he remained in coma and near coma. He had not been able to speak a single word during this period, nor had his consciousness cleared enough for him to signal us in any way. His only communication, if it were indeed that, had been agitation and pulling at his IVs and intubation equipment. I looked down at him in that hospital bed, small, frail, emaciated. He was at the mercy not only of his disease but of his oblivious, apathetic mother and the medical system: a system that could neither cure him nor grant him a dignified death. It was heartbreaking.

LOUIS BRYAN AND ALLEN DAY
DINNER PARTIES DWINDLE

I first met Louis Bryan in San Francisco in 1984 while in town for an interview with CPMC. Louis—slender, intelligent, exceptionally articulate (he speaks with just a hint of the west Texas in which he grew up)—was 43 at the time. We soon became friends. Louis' partner, Allen Day, was fair complexioned with a blond, drooping mustache; he was an artist of extraordinary talent who worked in graphic design south of the city. Even though I wasn't looking to replace him, Allen nonetheless felt a mixture of jealousy and genuine dislike for me. In a way, it was no wonder as there was a chasm between my sensibilities and his. I happened to be visiting their apartment in the Castro one afternoon when Allen arrived, having just bought a pair of red tennis shoes. When asked if I liked them, I offered something non-committal. But then, not willing to let well enough alone, I let slip my true opinion, saying "Well, at least they must be comfortable." This only solidified his distaste for me. In spite of this, and other unintended insults, Allen was, over time, forgiving: he allowed me entry into his and Louis' group of close friends. This was quite the largesse as the two of them would create, on special occasions, lavish evening dinner parties for which Louis would prepare an extraordinary variety of gourmet foods.

After these dinners, during a happy time filled with discussion and humor, when the plates still sat on the table, our hosts would occasionally produce a small, clear plastic vial of cocaine. Carefully constructed to apportion a single "dose" at a time, the squat little bottle, the size of a man's thumb, was then passed, person to person, around the dining room table. The camaraderie I felt persisted long

ANDREW M. FAULK, M.D.

after any transient "buzz" from the bit of cocaine I inhaled. When our friends began to suddenly drop out of sight (only to appear later in obituaries), the *Weltanschauung* of living in San Francisco in the mid-1980s gave us a permission, as if one were needed, for such "debauchery."

Towards the end of these evenings, Allen would bring out his "Retirement Fund," his portfolio of remarkable drawings. He worked in many different styles and techniques and never drew a face the same way twice. His collection was large and he believed that, when the day came for him to retire, these images would generate sufficient money, if not to live comfortably, at least to cover his needs. In the end, however, Allen wasn't to need any retirement portfolio.

There came a time when those faces around the dining room table became fewer and fewer; somber, empty chairs growing in number until the dinners ended entirely. It was in the middle of February, 1987, during my last year of residency, that Louis called me. He was anxious and upset; Allen's speech had become nonsensical and he had stopped going to work. Spending more and more time in bed in full retreat, Allen had developed a dry cough and a fever. Could I come over right away? When I arrived, I was struck by the uneasy mood in their grey Victorian house. As is so often the case in California, the contrast between the bright afternoon sunshine outside and the dark shadows within were disconcerting. I walked into Allen's bedroom and marked the difference between the gaunt form lying in front of me and the dinner party host of the past. He was emaciated with painfully thin extremities, sunken eyes and concave cheeks; AIDS-associated seborrheic dermatitis crevassed his face with red, flaking patches—all hallmarks of advanced HIV infection.

I sat down next to him on the bed. "How're you feeling?" I asked. Despite my walking into the room with Louis, Allen was surprised to see me. Between coughing jags he reported "I'm okay. These Twix candy bars are really great. You should try them." He handed me a candy bar. I didn't need to ponder; I asked Louis to follow me into the kitchen. "Louis," I said, "we need to get him to a hospital. It looks bad." Having seen other manifestations of AIDS and cognizant of the never-ending midnight in which we lived, Louis was, sadly, not surprised. It was no great emergency, so we got into my car for the short drive to CPMC. One look at the diffusely, whited-out X-ray of his lungs confirmed that it was almost certainly *Pneumocystis*. We began treating his pneumonia immediately—although I had my suspicions that more was involved. A severe infection can affect mental capacity, of course, but Allen's cognition seemed more compromised than usual for a 45-year-old man with pneumonia. There was a three-day wait for MRIs, but I knew the radiology technicians well and they scheduled a head MRI the afternoon of my request. It showed multiple sites of pathology consistent with *Toxoplasmosis*—an infectious disease in the immunocompromised and usually deadly for those with AIDS. We started him on antibiotics and Allen fully recovered from his PCP, but his brain *Toxoplasmosis* proved less easy to control and he never regained full mental capacity.

Allen and Louis had owned their house on Scott Street with a third investor. Fearing that Allen's biological family might compel a sale after his death that would force Louis out of his home, the two men bought Allen out. As marriage was illegal, financial arrangements and maneuvers such as this were common during those years—as were, unfortunately, last-minute changes in wills in which long-standing commitments and choices were changed and loved ones excluded to the benefit of genetic families. Allen's relationship with Louis and the extraordinary attention which Louis gave him during his last months were, however, understood and appreciated by Allen's family. In fact Allen's mother and Louis maintained a relationship until she died in 2012. This was unlike many other families who appeared oblivious to the vigilant care provided by the partner of their son, brother or father.

But like the majority of blood families I knew, Allen's was unwilling to disclose the true cause of his death. Ironically, had more families disclosed these diagnoses, perhaps there would have been a greater outcry for research and care. Quite probably the word "AIDS" might not have continued to carry its devastating stigma. Secrecy strangled advancement in investigation and acceptance. Instead Allen's mother told her people that he had died of a brain tumor. Allen was hospitalized twice more in those six months before he stepped off the earth. That August we lost yet another friend.

RICK
LEARNING NOT TO ASK

During my early years at Columbia University in New York, I had struck up a friendship with Bill Kellerman, a smart, well-educated stockbroker who lived in San Francisco. Years after I met him, I was to see him again in California.

Bill had a two-bedroom apartment near the Castro. It was sometime in the late 1980s that he offered to rent his extra bedroom to a young man named Rick who had hit a rough patch in his finances. He had reason to step into Rick's room one day and he noticed a stack of lined paper which was so uniform that Bill initially thought it was fresh from a stationary store. But on top of the stack, he found in a neat, cursive script a page with the sentence, "I am a good person. I will not get AIDS." The sentence was repeated again and again all the way to the bottom of the page. Bill lifted the page to see the next one underneath. It, too, had the same note carefully repeated. A chill went down Bill's spine. He checked the next page, and the next, and the next. Each page down to the bottom of the stack was covered with the same two sentences: "I am a good person. I will not get AIDS."

This, it seemed to me, was a testament to the terror, desperation and magical thinking of the time. When science is near helpless, and the disease is as lethal as AIDS, it is no wonder that some people embraced their atavistic impulses and turned toward amulets and incantations, shamans and witch doctors.

Rick moved out of Bill's apartment and I didn't hear of him for a year and a half. When he eventually came to mind and I inquired about him, Bill said he'd heard Rick had committed suicide a few months earlier. It was this kind of answer, repeated over and over, which led me to stop asking about people. And so I cultivated a fortress mentality: I stopped answering the phone, listening to phone messages and opening mail. I would tell myself that I would open the mail later, in a day or two, and it would stack, there on my living room coffee table, until the pile would become too unruly and spill over onto the floor. Eventually I would gather my strength, prepare for another death and open all the potential bomblets at once. But my system—if you can call it that—frequently failed and an envelope would go missing only to be found months later or sometimes not at all. Although I am improving, to this day I still find myself unable to immediately open unidentified mail or voice-mail when I suspect emotional content—I tell myself I'll open it when I am feeling stronger… and prepared.

JACK SOEHLKE
COMEDIAN AND SPOUSE

I met John Robert Soehlke, Jack to everyone, in the summer of 1987. I was preparing for the Board exam in Internal Medicine, but had gone out one night to the Eagle bar in San Francisco. (It seems most cities have a gay bar named the Eagle; if one wants to find a gay bar in an unknown city, one need only look for one called the Eagle.)

Jack was a remarkable person with a staggering sense of comedy that, more often than not, took the form of physical humor. He stood about 5'8" with a small frame and an oversized grin. It was a ready smile, but not an "easy" one as there was effort in his enthusiasm which was, nonetheless, quick and undiluted. His skin had that tawny southern European hue but his last name, Soehlke, belied the Italian heritage he claimed—although, of course, surnames and ancestry don't run as parallel as they did a hundred years ago. He walked quickly, but with many extra steps as he backtracked and re-checked whatever task took up his attention in the moment. In less formal settings, his speech was punctuated by the squeals and tonal rises at the end of sentences normally associated with the hypothetical questions of old-fashioned "school marms" and some of our more flamboyant brothers—or as poking fun at both. His comic instincts were accurate but he was perfectly aware of the emotional temperature of his surroundings.

Jack was one of the few people I have known who was capable of joy, not just happiness, but joy. With that quality came an ambition and ability to inspire it among those around him. He didn't have the intellectual underpinnings to be especially witty with words or ideas, for his humor was of a physical kind like that of Charlie Chaplin or Groucho Marx. He reproduced personality quirks and physical mannerisms of those around him with both hilarity and warmth. As with the great comedians, he would take a physical feature, usually kinetic, and reproduce it in an exaggerated, wonderfully entertaining, fashion. Much to the consternation of those around him unused to his ways, Jack would walk pretend stairs, tussle with imaginary crates and fight with unknown assailants. He would fall, convincingly, from unseen walls and mysterious precipices. He would struggle with mythical gates and argue with fabricated people. Sending museum guards into apoplexy, he would feign scratching a flake of paint off a priceless piece of art. He found his own performances delightful; I was charmed by their authenticity and audacity.

Jack used his voice as a major tool in his comedy and it went from a high-pitched giggle to deep and dramatic hyper-masculine speech. His imagination was not constrained by societal norms, and having an exceptionally malleable face, he could instantly turn a sympathetic or blank look into a mask of unbounded disbelief, unbridled sadness or faux horror. I have never seen anyone, excepting professional actors, so able to produce the quivering chin and trembling lips of impending tears. Groucho Marx had nothing on Jack when it came to listening to someone in apparent deep sincerity and then turning away from his "target" to express either total disbelief or pure revulsion. He didn't keep it a secret from those who knew him when he was listening to something absurd from a speaker out of his depth or out of his mind. Because of his sense of humor, his mother judged him trivial and unmanly. I knew better.

But Jack had another quieter, supportive side, characterized by an attentive focus on others. Just as he wanted to entertain others, he wanted to care for others, and perhaps that's really the same thing. He treated others, and certainly me, with thoughtfulness and generosity. For years after Jack's death, my parents, who had visited us in spite of some lingering qualms about my spiritual positioning, repeatedly remarked on his shouldering my care. I especially remember how it was after we moved to Los Angeles. It is difficult for me to explain my physical and mental state when I arrived home from work in those days. Jack would retrieve a soda from the refrigerator and say little but "hello." I would climb the stairs, then, of our two-story condo, shut the door to my study, and sit for a while in complete silence to decompress from the emotional concussions of the day—the

ANDREW M. FAULK, M.D.

discouraging defeats, the never-ending explanations, the inspiring courage, the heart-breaking tragedies. Although I managed them as best as I was able, these matters were not, could not, be resolved in a few hours or days, months or even years. I believed that there were too many patients to see, tests to review and hospital visits to make to grieve each loss. In the same way as I was to handle my mail years later, I thought I could postpone sorrow until I felt stronger and more able. It was a time when I assumed emotional shut-down of some kind was the lone option—compartmentalization, the sole choice. It was the only way I thought I could do what I did.

All the while I was struggling to suppress the turmoil of my own HIV. After an hour or so of preparing myself for a night of refuge, I would come back downstairs and there would be Jack: cheerful, innocent of the day's burdens and ignorant of my precarious journey through emotional chaos. His lightness balanced my heaviness. Had I helped calm one patient's titanic rage at the husband by whom she had been infected? Jack pretended he needed assistance to boil water. Had I broken the news to Richard Speakman that he was HIV-positive? Jack feared his risotto was something useful only to NASA.

Rarely did I ever tell him the details of my work. He loved me, but could not provide intellectual solace. Yet Jack's comic relief did worlds to knit my shattered pieces back together. No matter the steady drumbeat of approaching calamity—the perpetual, random loss of friends and patients—Jack had the talent to create a change in my reference point. His excitement was irrepressible as he welcomed me home for the trial run of his new little fountain in our tiny backyard. He was unsuccessfully "teaching" the puppy to heel by merely repeating the word "heel." Whether he was the comedian or the devoted spouse, he scattered tranquility as though he were a farmer seeding his fields.

For some time after our move to L.A., I was irritated by his lack of a job, but I soon came to rely on his care and humor and my annoyance lifted. He was employed for a short time as a perfume "sprayer" at the entrance to a large department store in the local mall and, while it lasted, I'd receive reports of celebrity spotting and shopper disagreements which were made all the more entertaining by Jack's delivery. And when that job became too boring and unfulfilling and he returned to full-time homemaking, I was still regaled by stories. Now they centered on Tina Turner's sister (who lived in our complex) as well as the eccentricities of our other neighbors, which also included a policeman and a dancer for an aging movie star. Jack always had some piece of diversion for me, and I began to count on him more and more. Despite my anxieties and idiosyncrasies, he loved taking care of me. At work I dealt with the sick and the suffering, the desperate and the dying, and at night he did his best to wash away my discouragement and exhaustion. His efforts found a ready audience in me and I came home every night with gratitude and, I pray now, with acknowledgment. He was a balance in our home for my heavy heart.

THE SYMBOL OF COMMITMENT

In October of 1989, Jack and I took a vacation to Germany, Austria and Italy and it was there in Venice that I bought his ring. But before that, before my birthday, we visited Salzburg. Jack's favorite movie was *The Sound of Music* and even at home he would sometimes break into its trademark "The hills are alive..." in an exaggerated, overly-dramatic falsetto which was hilarious to hear coming from a grown man. While in Salzburg we discovered there was a *Sound of Music* tour which included a distant look at the historical Von Trapp home and some sites made famous by the film. I was a little embarrassed to go on such a commercialized, saccharine-infused tour which ran counter to my natural reserve. But Jack was delighted that such a tour existed and, once this came to light, there was absolutely no doubt we would be taking it.

Once aboard *The Sound of Music* tour bus, by Jack's choice we sat in the front row. I discovered, to my chagrin, that the bus was principally peopled by older women. We were the youngest wayfarers and the only other male was someone we assumed to be a husband who appeared disgruntled and mortified. I myself wasn't as disgruntled as I was mortified, but I reasoned this was all due to my unattractive proclivity for occasional pretentiousness and that the tour should be appreciated for what it was. Such enjoyment, however, took time for me to cultivate and in the meantime my feelings swung between the cousins of embarrassment and humiliation. Shortly after the bus pulled away from the tourist depot, I was horrified to hear coming in chorus from the seat next to me the opening words: "The hills are alive..." I slowly sank into my seat to appear as small as possible. But to my surprise, as Jack continued to sing the soaring, iconic song of *The Sound of Music*, from the back of the bus I began to hear others join along. Soon, the entire bus was singing "I go to the hills, when my heart is lonely..." There was nothing I could do, I was captive and my resistance was melting. "To sing through the night, like a lark who is learning to pray," I warbled. At the conclusion, irrepressible Jack began to sing it again in case anyone had missed out on a chorus.

During that trip to Europe we found ourselves in Venice, without planning, on my birthday. Walking down one of the narrow streets, we stumbled upon a small jewelry store in which we found a simple zircon ring of deep yellow gold, more yellow, we were told, than the gold that is sold in the US. Much of Jack's charm rose from his instant enthusiasm for various people and places and he immediately fell in love with the ring. Jack was not a man frequently drawn to physical objects, however, which made gift-giving occasions difficult, but knowing that this would make him happy, the ring was a windfall for me. I had discovered something which would please him and something that was a universal symbol of love and attachment. In 1989 marriage equality wasn't on the horizon and domestic partnership legalities weren't even in our consciousness, so a ring was the closest we came to symbolized commitment. By way of diversion, however, I told him that I didn't think as much of the ring as he did and that we couldn't afford it anyway. We walked back to our hotel for a mid-afternoon nap and I could tell the ring was on his mind. On arriving the concierge handed the key to Jack, who promptly pretended to drop it. We searched but I knew the location of the room key was not the mystery it seemed. Jack spent several minutes looking around the floor, even bringing in innocently helpful, hapless strangers until he "discovered" it. The concierge, who seemed to quickly catch on, wasn't entertained—but I was.

Up in the room, I pretended to nap while Jack furtively slipped outside. Once he was gone, I raced to the jewelry store and bought the gold ring. Hoping to reach the hotel before he could return, I ran along the narrow, confusing streets. But Jack and I both reached the entrance to the hotel at the same time and both pretended that running into each other was expected. As if supplementary excursions were part of our tour, neither of us attempted an explanation. In his hands he carried an Italian version of a birthday cake and in my back pocket I carried the gold ring. That night, at some Venetian restaurant, we presented each other with our gifts. One of my cherished memories is of Jack's response: his smile sparkled more than usual and lasted throughout dinner and the walk home. And in the morning it was as bright as the night before.

After returning to the States I had the zircon exchanged for a diamond. Jack was so pleased that eventually it took a jeweler's warning before he halted the repetitive polishing of the ring; the setting would disappear, after all, if polished to excess.

SQUINT YOUR EYES

While Jack was without a full-time job when we met in San Francisco in 1987, he usually worked as a distributor of low-end perfumes and occasionally as a window dresser for various department stores. But I think the work he enjoyed the most was arranging flowers. We'd been dating for a number of months when he got a job arranging flowers for a friend's wedding in Los Gatos, which is about an hour south of the city. In that deadly serious tone of his, which was often followed by a high-pitched giggle, he reminded me about his technique for evaluating his various bouquets, "Now you have to squint your eyes and look at the entire arrangement to really appreciate the colors and pattern!" Turning toward his creations at the front of the church, by way of example, he peered through lids squeezed nearly shut. Squinting your eyes and looking at the whole, I thought, was his philosophy of life—a philosophy I could deeply appreciate. After the wedding was over and the clean-up finished, we headed back to San Francisco with Jack driving my car while I napped in the passenger seat.

After arriving back in the city, we spent the night in my apartment. He had had a dry cough for the preceding two days and I still can't understand why it didn't dawn on me that there was a problem. At around 2 a.m. I was awakened by his coughing and shortly afterwards he began to develop "air hunger" which was ominous. I read his temperature which was a startling 102.5 degrees and took out my stethoscope and listened to his lungs; my heart sank when I heard a bilateral ("double") pneumonia. He almost certainly had PCP. Although a pneumonia was disconcerting, the implication it conveyed was devastating—Jack was immunocompromised: he had HIV. He was dying and I felt I barely had had the chance to get to know him. And could I, was I prepared to, walk him down that path? Time and again I had seen the consequences of caring for someone who was dying of the illness. We had only been dating for a short time and it would have been understandable had I ended our relationship then. I had previously told myself, considering what I had seen and knowing what I knew, that I wouldn't get involved with anyone facing end-stage AIDS; the stress involved would accelerate the progression of my own disease. But he and I had clicked in a beautiful way and I never seriously considered breaking off the relationship.

As Jack didn't know, and didn't want to know, his HIV status, we had conducted our relationship carefully. It was my policy to strongly encourage everyone to be tested, but I didn't pressure my patients. I knew full well how devastating it could be to learn one's status and I trusted my men to know what was best for themselves. It was a trade-off: knowing one's status could give one early warning of opportunistic diseases and make anything but safe sex radioactive, but if constant stress was the result, the education would speed one's immune system collapse. Whether or not a patient agreed to the test, I vigorously pushed safe sex strategies such as not having sex while high and placing condoms in strategic locations—no matter how unlikely the setting. Obviously I could not have been more forceful in condemning the use of needles, sterilized or not. There was also another significant disincentive to have one's HIV status checked: insurance companies, whether medical or life, could demand patient disclosure. Should one lie, should information be revealed at some future date, the insurance companies pledged to refuse to honor such a claim. The homicidal insurance companies were nothing if not shrewd. (It is not paranoid to be wary of submitting one's genetic profile in ancestry pursuit, as repurposing tests for one's medical susceptibilities would allow insurance companies to similarly take one's oath hostage.)

Jack had had a previous partner, Ted, who had been hyper-vigilant for any newly-appearing signs of AIDS, especially Kaposi's Sarcoma. His maniacal inspections had been pointless for he died from AIDS anyway. During those years having paranoia about one's health may have been pointless, but it wasn't unusual. We were, after all, in the Dark Ages.

In carrying out the logistics for Jack's hospitalization, I buried my emotions, for I believed that my feelings had to be "postponed." As would happen time and again later in my medical career, dealing with my emotions in the moment was an expenditure of time and energy I believed I could not afford. Now I understand that even in the worst of circumstances, even when emotional catastrophe seems too overwhelming to be processed immediately, sorrow is best experienced at the time of loss; delay only inflicts greater psychological cost. But surprising as it may sound, at the age of 33, I was still a child when it came to coping with such feelings. I can't judge myself too harshly, though, for shutting down emotionally in an attempt to postpone grief is a natural human reaction. It is almost instinctive to take a course which may seem less painful in the moment when the option of a choice isn't evident—to accidentally stumble onto a route which cloaks a hidden cost. For a kernel of my grief was, of course, sorrow for my own losses: every relationship, every success, every passion, every dream was to be taken from me. Not in the distant future, not after 40 or 50 years, but soon. I had moved from a point in life where I was no longer experiencing the accumulating years of youth, but the subtractions of an older age I had not yet attained.

I drove Jack to CPMC where a friend in radiology agreed to do a chest X-ray off-record. Afterwards, as Jack waited in the radiology anteroom, I threw his chest film onto a light box and flipped it on. My heart sank—the film showed his lungs were whited out with the dense infiltrates of PCP. I felt as if I'd had the breath smacked out of me.

The experience of suddenly knowing my partner's diagnosis would be repeated 14 years later. In March 2002, Lance Newman (my future partner) was admitted to the University of California San Francisco hospital with chest pain. There, too, I learned the gravity of his condition before he did. In the ER with Lance, I looked over the shoulder of the technician taking the 12-lead EKG and was shocked to see not only evidence of ongoing cardiac ischemia (oxygen deficiency) but also indications of a "completed" heart attack sometime in the past. In both cases, I had the information before they did and my partners were more ill than they knew. It is common sense that physicians shouldn't treat their own families. Even when the doctor isn't the physician for the family member, it is tricky. Sometimes bad news is best given by a family member, sometimes not. Occasionally in a patient's mind, the physician is associated with the illness and so it may be best to be on the patient's "side" of the diagnosis. It may happen that a doctor who is also the significant other might be uncomfortable responding to an avalanche of questions. In these particular doctor-patient equations, I felt it was important that I stood with them and that they be informed by their own physician, not me. My responsibility was to reassure them both, to reveal as little by voice or facial expression as possible before their own doctors told them their condition. I was a physician, but I wasn't *their* physician.

In case my examination of Jack at home, and the ubiquity of HIV, had not revealed the diagnosis, his chest X-ray did. He had received the AIDS' death sentence and it was up to his physician to determine how the information should be presented. But here, I reasoned, distance was difficult to maintain when AIDS was so well known. I decided to say what I usually said in similar circumstances: I told him it looked like PCP but that we needed more information for a final diagnosis.

As he didn't have medical insurance, I knew CPMC couldn't care for him and I would need to drive him to San Francisco General where those without insurance could receive care. Thankfully, I could step back.

We arrived at San Francisco General, and I stood by his side while he was admitted through the ER, a task made simpler and faster by the X-ray I held in my hands. He had a habit of "clucking" his tongue in a sound that communicated "this is the way it is—nothing can be done about it." It was to be a night filled with clucking. My emotions grew numb as a psychological distance between me and the information began to form. Although he took the diagnosis well, he knew what it meant. We didn't know how long he had; we didn't know how long any of us had. But in that uncertainty was a bit of hope.

As we worked through admission and the beginning of treatment, his clucking intensified, but I saw quiet courage as I would see it in so many others and it is what I hope to demonstrate when I approach my last hours. Bravery is confronting danger and pain without feeling fear; courage is facing those hurdles despite fear. The essence of courage is not the absence of fear—it is the presence of fear, the understanding of the consequences and the deliberate choice to fight. I have never promised anyone a particular response when it comes to my own final illness—it may be hostility or rage. Or serenity and productive reflection. I believe that I know too much to be brave; that my experiences have come to rest in my DNA.

The question was not if we were to die—we are all destined to die. Rather it was when, the question was how soon. As if in battle, bombs were raining all around and we knew at any moment, without warning, we could be annihilated. Like those next to us, each day could be our last. Unlike a war zone, however, when our brothers stepped off the earth, there was no deafening explosion or cratered earth; our men went quietly to their graves. It seemed wrong for a life filled with talk and laughter, song and shouting, to end with only the quiet murmur of a faint exhale.

VIV AND GUS SOEHLKE
NO HELP FROM THE PARENTS

Jack asked that I call his parents, Gus and Viv, and tell them he had a serious pneumonia. They lived in Collinsville, Illinois, a suburb of St. Louis, and this was to be my first interaction with his parents. It did not go well. It quickly became apparent that his mother was more concerned about who had "given" him the disease than the details of his diagnosis and prognosis. As I was on the phone reporting his illness, I instantly became an easy target for her confusion and anger. I had given HIV to Jack, she concluded—in effect, I had taken a gun and shot her son dead. Unfortunately that was to set the tone of our relationship as her grief spun into ever increasing anger. But her overall response wasn't entirely anger at me; Viv was also angry with Jack. It was obvious that she believed his behavior had been irresponsible and he deserved his illness. It was a reaction I heard many times from many others who didn't recognize that truth: only one exposure to one person was all that was necessary for infection. Of course it was easy to condemn gay men with HIV, for their sexual activity itself, already a preoccupation of the heterosexual world, was considered repugnant. Sometimes she communicated her disgust in words and sometimes just in her tone of voice. It was an ugly way of dealing with the disease and sometimes came from family members who had never accepted their son, father or brother's sexual orientation to begin with.

That first day in the hospital, when Jack was formally diagnosed with PCP, I was bending over him with my stethoscope listening to his heart, when he breathed a very audible wheeze. I showed no outward sign of hearing the abnormality. He, on the other hand, reacted to it: his face contorted not into a mask of heartbreak or horror, but rather into a facetious register of contrived alarm and sham distress. Imagine, not fear and despair, but faux devastation in a hospital room! But it was Jack's nature to bypass these reactions with a humor born from detached amusement and an optimism of unknown origin. Although there were many other reasons, I loved him for this.

I went home that night exhausted. I had slept little in the chair next to his bed the night before and I had to return to work the next day. In spite of his parents' judgmental reaction, they remained much of the week before flying back to Illinois. But I was correct in my immediate take that they would not be helping me handle Jack's condition. Viv, it seemed, lived in a state of constant anger. She was angry long before his diagnosis and would remain so, I believed, long after he passed away. Her hostile attitude was to show up repeatedly. Once, when I took them out to dinner in Collinsville, she deftly turned my victory into defeat when she complained about the salad and accused the restaurant of adding sugar. Later she announced to the restaurant at large that the smells emanating from the fish at the next table were making her nauseous. So it was a frosty reception I received when they first entered his hospital room that day. Jack's father, Gus, took most of his cues from Viv, but he nevertheless treated Jack with a compassion that Viv's anger would not allow. Being a retired high school gym instructor, he coached Jack with the tools he had, suggesting that physical exercises would speed up healing. Gus gave what he could and performed examples of his exercises. Although his naïveté may have been painful to watch, his loving contribution was deeply moving. Jack, however, clucked his tongue so often that week that even he noticed it, but it was a compulsion he could not control.

In spite of my own opinion of the emotional state of his parents, I realized that, for my sake, things would go better if I allowed them some forgiveness. He was their son, after all, and they were as upset and afraid as I was.

After recovering from his bout with PCP, Jack did remarkably well on *Pneumocystis* prophylaxis and the heavy, usually debilitating, doses of azidothymidine (AZT) prescribed at the time. His energy and outlook remained at their usual high. Approaching death was on his mind, of course, but he rarely discussed this, nor allowed fear or self-pity to overwhelm him. He knew, however—we both knew—that his final illness was inevitable and, in all probability, soon. We were wrong, as he was not diagnosed with AIDS-related Non-Hodgkin's Lymphoma until late 1990 and lived until 1991.

JOHN LORE, M.D. AND JIM CARLTON, M.D.
STARTING A PRACTICE

After graduating from my Internal Medicine Residency at CPMC in 1987, I was the only one of my class to be asked to join an established medical practice in town. In the end this was to prove a mixed blessing. I was to take the place of Wayne Bolles, M.D., a retiring doctor in Dr. Jim Carlton's office, which would formally link up with Dr. John Lore's practice. James Carlton had a growing HIV practice which was expanding daily as the epidemic ballooned around us; the ever-growing numbers overwhelmed him with a workload that had become unmanageable. Both physicians were gay and I was excited; I could finally come out in my profession! After years of carefully maintaining my professional closet, I could finally bulldoze its walls and set fire to the remains. But the potential legal ramifications remained, however, and my HIV status had to remain a secret, even from my eventual colleagues at Lawrence Medical in Los Angeles. But, for the first time in medicine, I no longer needed to hide my sexual orientation. I felt such incredible freedom!

Jim Carlton was the classic image of the absent-minded professor: even his gait was tentative as he'd stop-and-start as he alternated between talking and thinking. Deep in thought, Jim always appeared to be lost even when I was certain he knew his location. John Lore was the more down-to-earth, nuts-and-bolts, entrepreneurially savvy of the two physicians. He was as sophisticated and polished as Jim Carlton was not. He laughed easily and knew exactly what to say to put patients and their families at ease and inspire trust and confidence. Though Carlton and Lore were an unlikely pair, they were equal in the quality of care they delivered to their patients;

each was an academic and consistently up-to-date in his knowledge of diagnoses and treatments. With our new association, John Lore moved his office space next door to Jim Carlton's. There was much discussion as to how to combine the two disparate populations— Carlton's practice being young men who clearly had AIDS (perhaps emaciated, coughing, with visible KS lesions) and Lore's practice was a mixture of older women and up-and-coming professionals. We carefully strategized the best way to preserve both practices and make the waiting rooms comfortable for both sets of patients. John Lore moved his practice next door to Jim Carlton's which gave me access to two waiting rooms: Lore's was reserved for the non-HIV patients and Carlton's for the growing HIV population. Such was the temperament of the times that two separate waiting rooms seemed the best way to make both groups comfortable and a practice viable.

GENERAL DOROTHY
OVERBOOKING AND BOOKKEEPING

Unfortunately for my career in San Francisco, my relationship with their receptionist, Dorothy, had quickly soured after my practice began. Dorothy, dressed in a nurse's uniform complete with white cardboard tiara, with no more than a high school education, reigned from our front waiting room, which also served as her office. It seemed that she spent much of her time painting over charting mistakes with "white out." She made my days with Carlton and Lore an embarrassment that blossomed into a nightmare. From my office I could hear her on the phone giving patients badly-flawed recommendations which were distressingly dangerous. Once during a pelvic exam, with my patient full in the table stirrups, Dorothy had interrupted by banging on the door and loudly insisting I come out immediately to attend to a hospitalized patient. Dorothy constantly spoke to me as if she were the responsible physician and I was the untutored receptionist. In fact Dorothy spoke to both Carlton and me as if we were delinquent children. To see my patients' reactions to her condescending abuse was not only distressing but fraught with potential consequence; if the receptionist-secretary needed to "manage" me this way, could patients be expected to trust me?

As I had purchased the part of the practice that belonged to Dr. Wayne Bolles, I was gradually paying him slowly decreasing percentages of my earnings. After my payments to Bolles, however, I was barely making more than parking expenses in the downtown San Francisco building which also housed our offices. As my schedule in the Carlton/Lore office was constantly full, rough calculations of what my pay should have been was beginning to make me wonder if Dorothy was practicing some creative bookkeeping—doctor offices are famous for staff embezzlement. Two years after I left the practice, Dorothy's machinations saw daylight. The IRS knocked on my door with not one but two errant "W-2s." Evidently she had been generously helping herself to the office till while attributing her extra income to me and gifting me with the tax bill. The police told me that should I want justice, I would need to have an attorney intervene. I paid the taxes with interest and fines.

Throughout my career I've tried to keep my patients' appointments and have them wait as little as possible—this is, hopefully, the goal of every physician. But some offices double-book their patients to prevent any unproductive "down time." This was not my particular style and I informed Dorothy of this fact. Nevertheless she repeatedly overbooked me. When I drew her attention to her disturbing scheduling, she said that this was Dr. Bolles' way of doing things. And then, as was her custom, she looked down, opened a desk drawer and took out her bottle of white out; our conversation was over. With all that was going on in my life—Jack's diagnosis, pandemonium in the office, Dorothy's autocratic inflexibility, two separate waiting rooms with two different sets of patients, my own HIV status and, most importantly, patient care—some days I was running on fumes. I needed to present myself to my patients as calm and confident; I needed to *be* calm and confident. I needed some tranquility in my life.

You don't get if you don't ask.

My attempt to insist on office changes went badly and I watched as the proverbial car crashed. Out of the office, on the tiny back deck of my small apartment, I told Jim Carlton of my problems with Dorothy. Jim Carlton's response was not only dismissive but also revealed unwanted Freudian insight into his curious mentality. He responded to my complaints, "Oh, if you think she's hard to live with, you should have been around my mother." I was astonished! His extraordinarily inappropriate response was outrageous on so many levels. It was an indication of my naïveté that I thought any other response was possible when I questioned her finances and gave Jim the ultimatum that either she or I leave the office, he took not a heartbeat to thank me for my time working in their office.

Parenthetically, in spite of the indignity of his instant choice of the madwoman Dorothy, I will always have a soft spot for the painfully insecure and voluntarily-abused Jim Carlton. Whenever I phoned Jim's home, I would hear another man's voice on his answering machine. Upon questioning John Lore about this, he told me that it was the voice of Jim's partner who had died long ago—it was a recording Jim couldn't bring himself to erase and replace with his own message. This was not unusual: across the city telephones were being answered with the voices of long-passed lovers. The day before Jack died, I myself recorded a new greeting over the endearingly playful message Jack had recorded—I knew once he was gone I'd never have the strength to erase the message I'd come to know intimately and love dearly.

I ESCAPE THE PROFESSIONAL CLOSET

Throughout my residency and internship at CPMC, there were, as there always are, references in records and people's remarks about other doctors, former doctors. On questioning I would hear the names and short stories of other gay M.D.s who had died from AIDS. As was routine back in those days, you learned of others' passing in short asides.

"Oh, Doctor X, I don't see him caring for so-and-so anymore."

"Yes, he passed away last year."

"Really? How old was he?" (Don't we always question the ages of the deceased to compare ourselves to those who have passed? If they're younger, or just plain young, we press to know details. Could we be subject to a similar twist of fate?)

"I don't know, early thirties I'd guess. AIDS got him." These were the ghosts of former physicians and many of these names and faces, even after the passing of time, I remember clearly. As time progressed, however, the names of these earlier physicians who had passed were heard less often, only to be eclipsed by the newer names of those more recently lost.

After I'd finished the residency requirements for Board Certification in Internal Medicine, the necessary examination followed. In order to prepare, I signed up for a one week Internal Medicine review class in San Diego. In classrooms people often sit in the same seats, day after day, and I was no exception; each day found me close to the front. During the course there were multiple occasions when the reviewer asked a question and the audience was given the chance to answer. I found myself comparing whispered answers with a nattily-dressed physician sitting next to me. I happened to answer many of these questions correctly—the gentleman sitting next to me, not as frequently. As the week progressed, I began to eat lunch with him and we exchanged our personal stories. Vincent Briar, M.D. had already taken the exam a surprising number of times but had yet to pass. He was in practice with Fred Lawrence, M.D. in Los Angeles; together they formed a partnership, Lawrence Medical Group, which was made up of the two of them, two physician assistants and a psychologist.

On Thursday of this week-long review, at lunch Vincent Briar, M.D. asked me if I were gay. My work in the Lore/Carlton office had not yet begun and my historic policy remained in place: no professional disclosure until I passed the Medical Board exam. I told him no, I wasn't gay.

"Although I'm straight, I work in a gay practice with primarily gay patients. For us, sexual orientation is not an issue," Vincent informed me.

That night I went back to the hotel and pondered what I had said. I debated with myself throughout the evening—Vincent's question, of course, had been an innocent one. Certainly my years in pre-med classes left me with an abiding sense of vulnerability and, though the ridiculous tie-cutting imbroglio with Dr. LeFou at the UW had nothing to do with my sexual orientation, it reinforced a sense of easy replacement and casual substitution.

But the winds of change were blowing across the country and I was just one exam away from Board Certification. All the intense years of medical school, internship and residency were behind me. I realized that I was no longer professionally vulnerable; whatever this stranger from L.A. thought of me would not impact my final goal. The next day, Friday, was the last day of the course and at lunch I sheepishly told Vincent I was gay. I explained my reasoning and standing policy, although no explanation was needed for Vincent— he understood perfectly. He immediately offered me a position at Lawrence Medical which I declined; I already had a job with the newly-combined practice of John Lore and Jim Carlton. He told me to keep his offer in mind, however, and we exchanged business cards.

Although I'd had a logical and understandable policy in place, it was time for it to be discarded, time for me to come out of my carefully constructed closet. It took some courage to identify myself fully to Dr. Briar, but the redemption made it worthwhile and was a taste of the professional freedoms to come.

It was months later, after I had been driven nearly insane by Dorothy's monarchy, that I resigned—disregarding the common sense rule that one should never abandon a job without another in hand. It was precisely the last day of my tenure at the Dr. Carlton/ Mother Dorothy circus that I got Vincent's call from L.A. He had an HIV patient relocating to San Francisco—could I follow him?

"No, Vincent, I can't help you," I said, "I won't be in practice here anymore." I summarized Dorothy's imperial behavior and Jim's response to my naïve "her or me" ultimatum.

Once again Vincent Briar offered me a job on the spot.

FRED LAWRENCE, M.D.
THINKING LARGE

I had initially refused Vincent Briar's early offers to join Lawrence Medical in Los Angeles; my wounds were still fresh from the Lore/ Carlton debacle. How could I be sure I wasn't walking into another office with behavioral and ethical problems? Besides, I didn't want to leave a city that had made itself a unique home for gay people, Bohemians, and misfits, a haven of political and sexual tolerance. San Francisco had been my first exposure to California and, besides its unconventional citizens, I was hypnotized by the foggy weather and surrounding natural beauty. (This was before the turn of the last century after which it became significantly larger and substantially different.) I saw L.A., on the other hand, as its famous cliché—a sweltering, intellectual wasteland consumed by superficial appearance and political apathy. Mistaking my snobbery and suspicion for strategy, Briar offered more incentive: he suggested a trial run. For working in L.A. one week a month, the practice would pay me the equivalent of a month's work in San Francisco plus airfare to Los Angeles and back. It was a plan that sounded perfect for me; soon I was working at the LMG office and flying back and forth between the two cities. Instead of General Dorothy, I discovered Rhonda, their chief receptionist. She was efficient, playful and had that sixth sense of knowing which situations required immediate attention. Their office was not only friendly and harmonious but also well-run. At the LMG office, staff called Fred Lawrence "doctor" as if the word "doctor" were a name itself. I thought this system was brilliant: this custom signaled everyone that Dr. Lawrence was a comrade, while still giving him respect and differentiation. (The practice couldn't

ANDREW M. FAULK, M.D.

extend to us, however—we were always "Dr. Briar" and "Dr. Faulk." After all, it would be confusing to have more than one physician in the office simply called "doctor.") Such efforts to create a healthy and satisfying work environment for everyone convinced me. Soon Jack and I were temporarily living in a small hotel in Hollywood.

Vincent rather than Fred had recruited me, so I first met Fred while he was house hunting in the Hollywood Hills. We met at the house he was examining that day which he found unacceptable. I, on the other hand, got a better review. In only a matter of months I was integrated into the efficient, happy staff of Lawrence Medical and Fred had found a quirky house on Outpost Drive which had been owned long before by a famous Hollywood film star of 1930s' horror movies. It was an extravagant affair with a small waterfall, holding pond, swimming pool, changing cabana and a concealed man-cave. The house was quirky, no doubt, but Fred was a match in eccentricity: at the Christmas parties held there every year it was expected that each of his guests would gift him with an item in silver.

It was appropriate that Fred Lawrence lived in the spotlight for he was larger than life. He was a force of nature who had achieved wealth and prestige by seizing opportunities that others either didn't see or didn't have the audacity to exploit. He thought large. The Roman philosopher Seneca said that luck is what happens when preparation meets opportunity. If that is so, Fred had done a lot of preparing and when it came to opportunities, Fred had usually created them too. With his imagination and abilities, he could transform a bad undertaking into a good one and, if that was not possible, discard it with speed and finesse. Fred saw expansion where others saw risk, bargains where others saw junk, and the gifted and capable where others saw the ordinary and troublesome.

Fred's practice included many of his personal friends that he had been seeing for years. He navigated these relationships, which can sometimes be problematic, with ease. Being friends with one's patients is optimum is so many ways. But this can be tricky for sometimes a patient associates their physician with whatever disease they may have and can therefore make him or her a target of misplaced anger and resentment. Also, as a near correlate, some interactions are best made by someone who is on the other side of the divide separating a patient from their physician. I am firmly opposed to ever lying to a patient but when Jack was a day before death and asked for the next move in his care, as his partner I lied to him. In this case, as I was not *his* physician, I was ethically comfortable with this particular deception. Had I been his physician I would at least have had an ethical struggle (although, even had this been the case, I probably would have set aside my routine sensibilities). But I knew him well, had struggled with him in his denial, and believed this was the right thing to do.

Sometime during the early 1970s Fred had been a *Playgirl* centerfold. At the time, he had such compelling good looks that the magazine had placed him front and center, literally. Oddly enough I had seen that particular issue in the '70s, though much later than its printing, lying about in the not-fit-for-rental apartment that my friend Norman Nash kept as his New York *pied-à-terre* on West 19th Street. But I saw the issue again during the course of my work at Lawrence Medical Group when Fred himself showed it to me. It was not that he left it lying about for the world to see. He had brought it into the office and, protecting it from any uninvited glance, showed it to me alone. Had I myself ever looked that becoming and received such exposure, I suspect the walls of my office, including the waiting room and patients' bathroom, would have been wallpapered with the issue.

Lawrence had been one of the very first physicians to advertise. His ads often took whole pages of the local gay rag and, later, smaller portions of national magazines. LMG regularly purchased entire tables at AIDS fund-raising events. He occasionally placed photos of us in these ads, so my face and specialized area of practice became somewhat recognizable in the community. As I was becoming known as an HIV physician, greeting a patient in the street might be an indication of someone's positive HIV status and so I never acknowledged a patient first. Without their greeting I behaved as if I'd never seen them. Not everyone understood this tactic, and it led some to conclude I was cold and aloof.

One of Fred's maxims was "punctuality is power" and that if one wished for a particular item or event, one had to be sitting at the table on time. After learning this, I was often early at morning meetings and became privy to remarks not necessarily intended for staff or peers. Despite his career he drove his Mercedes-Benz with the speed and abandon of a NASCAR 500 racer—clearly he liked to nurture a bad-boy image. Pam was his personal assistant as well as the glue holding together much of our practice. It was at several morning meetings that I heard Pam and him discuss his latest speeding ticket and the various penalties—such as traffic school—that he would be forced to endure.

Fred was a expensive dresser, with designer suits that fit him flatteringly. He ate almost exclusively at fine restaurants, usually with an entourage of several different people who orbited around him like so many planets around a star. In my time this included his interior decorator, a Frenchman, Jacques Charmant, who seemed to live with him on and off. In fact, for my parents' first visit to my new office in Los Angeles, we had met Fred in a trendy restaurant with a constellation of his subjects in full gravitational pull. In an over-the-top remark consistent with his style, he thanked my parents for birthing me, as I was "a gift to medicine" and certainly to his humble practice. Jacques, upon being introduced to my mother, kissed her outstretched hand which both surprised and charmed her. Fred was in his element.

CHRIS CARLEY
A CHAIR NEXT TO THE BED

In one of my first weeks in L.A., I saw patient Chris Carley. Among many innovations, Lawrence Medical had one custom that was incredibly helpful for patient care. Upon first being seen by the practice, the patient was photographed there at the front desk with the resulting Polaroid instant photo being attached to his chart. It was a terrific idea, giving doctors and staff an easy memory aid for telephone calls or M.D. "sign-offs" for night or week-end coverage. (Unfortunately, the patients with facial KS sometimes became so disfigured that even with photos, our staff had difficulty recognizing them.)

I recall his entering photo—Chris, blond, blue-eyed, looking young and robust at 30 and yet uncomfortable under the lens of the camera. I am not sure why I took a special interest in him—perhaps it was his quiet, introverted way or maybe his unassuming personality resonated with my own. As was the norm he had come in for his initial HIV results alone but as I got to know him he seemed socially isolated. Besides encouraging group therapy, Fred often recommended patients invest in a large TV. Frequently, as the disease progressed, watching TV became a patient's only entertainment and too often their only friend. For whatever reasons, perhaps partially due to the stigma of sexual orientation, many patients were without close friends or family which left them alone and lonely in darkened bedrooms with a TV their only company.

Chris asked for me on his return appointments and complained of very little during his office visits; his being seen was almost always for follow-up to monitor his health and determine if any new

ANDREW M. FAULK, M.D.

medication had been discovered to treat HIV. He seemed slightly more fearful than most patients I saw, but he carried it in a quiet way, without histrionics or morbid speculation. It was obvious he didn't enjoy being in an exam room, but he shouldered this discomfort in a workman-like way. Chris, like most patients in the practice, was usually seen alone and, despite the discomfort he felt being examined and discussing his illness, he seemed content in his isolation. That comfort in solitude seemed the most compelling characteristic he and I had in common.

As Chris' T-cells slipped lower and lower, it seemed to me that his isolation was more and more of an impediment and that his life would be prolonged, and happier, if there were someone providing some support. And as for my universal advice to "Get happy!" he seemed unable to do that. I sensed that others could provide a happiness, and of course support, that his routine solitude could not.

As his health deteriorated, I delved deeper into his social support. He had a mother living somewhere in the San Joaquin Valley of California but no father and no siblings; he seemed to have few, if any, friends. As the horizon of his life inched into view, I pushed him harder and harder to tell his mother, if no one else, of his HIV diagnosis. He resisted, and I should probably have seen that as evidence of a parent who was unable to help her son in any crisis. I was to discover in hindsight that involving his mother in his care was hardly the best answer for Chris' life.

If any one of my patients spoke of needing to tell their loved one or their family of their sexual orientation, I offered my help—far too many families learned at the bedside.

During one of our discussions, it seemed apparent that he was working out the end of his life alone. I pressed him to inform his mother. I said I would be happy to discuss the situation with her, in his presence, if he felt that might be helpful. He overcame his intuitive reluctance, finally, and came in with his mother. As they entered my exam room, he told me, under his breath, that he had disclosed his positive status to her just that morning. As I explained the medical situation and the unknown variables in his condition, she increasingly demonstrated a disturbing narcissism. Her questions revolved around herself and her own reaction to his illness, not to him or his ordeals. There, in front of him, she voiced her fears of what his illness would do to her and of how his orientation and disease made it impossible for her to inform those in her own social support network. When she began questioning infectivity and her own safety in being around her son, his eyes glazed over. Clearly, I had made a mistake in pushing him to bring his mother into the loop.

In January of 1991, my world was crumbling around me—by then, Fred Lawrence was ill and Jack was undergoing chemotherapy at the University of California Los Angeles (UCLA) hospital. Chris' downward spiral was another blow, albeit far lesser, to my psychological equilibrium. The last time I saw him he was hospitalized in a large room at the Medical Center of North Hollywood. Although the sun had set, the shades were drawn. The TV was off and his hospital tray stand had nothing on it except a styrofoam cup with a straw in it. The back of his bed was raised and there, silhouetted by the fluorescent light panel behind him, Chris sat in a space empty of sound and people and stared ahead into a vacant room and the desolate future before him.

He was bright enough to know medicine had little to offer beyond pain control, indeed he asked no questions about further treatment. Words failed in the tableau before me: offering hope to this man would have been an affront to his intelligence. My efforts to create a social structure to combat his isolation hadn't worked— the meeting with his mother had been a miserable failure. Despite opiates for his pain, he lay awake, mentally intact and aware of approaching death. In our last days, most of us fear pain and loss of personal autonomy, but he still had control of his bodily functions, so I asked him whether or not he was in pain. He replied no, but said nothing more. I couldn't read anything in his face and although I am comfortable with silence, the quiet here was agonizing. I was walking into a familiar situation, yet it was unfamiliar at the same time. Often, distant patients become surprisingly accessible when they're confronted with approaching death, but this was not to be Chris Carley's way. I began to see, however, that I didn't need to say anything profound. I could give him quite possibly the most important gift any of us can give the dying—our presence.

In those days, before the advent of laptop computers and digitized patient records, physicians would sit at the centralized nursing desks and write out in longhand reports of patients' progress and orders for tests and therapies. Nurses disliked any removal of patients' charts from their stations because their absence could be a source of escalating confusion. I understood; I appreciated the perennial need for a central location for information. But my connectedness with those in my care was paramount, and I felt it could best be obtained by charting in Chris' room. I gathered all the records of my various patients and moved them into his room, sat down in a chair next to his bed, and began the process of charting. I believe that my quiet presence next to my men provided what routine medical training and expertise could not.

When I charted in the hospital, I often would choose the patient who was the most ill or isolated and work in his room, next to his bed. Sometimes these patients were barely conscious, sometimes they were awake and talkative. Whether it was due to social abrasiveness, or perhaps conspicuous eccentricities, there were always some of my patients who had few social skills and fewer friends; it was not unusual for many to face their illness more or less alone. Although I needed quiet in which to write my notes and orders, this was usually an hour or so in which I could be a presence for my patients.

* * *

In spite of his debilitating macular degeneration, by the time my father passed at the age of 98 he had read this manuscript not once, but twice. This must have been quite the task for it was shortly after this he began to greet people not with his usual, cheerful "Hi! How are you?" but rather an equally bright "Hi! Who are you?!" However he had not, in fact, read this particular rendition—for I had given him a book edited specifically for him. In his particular version, I had carefully excised all the parts which I knew would trouble his sensibilities. It was this routine charting next to patients' beds which moved him the most for he frequently mentioned it to me and others.

GEORGE KRIVACEK AND LLOYD BURR
LIVING ON BORROWED TIME

It was during my first days in the HIV clinic, which Fred Lawrence had lovingly engineered, that I was introduced to George Krivacek, a long-standing patient. He was an immigrant from what was then Czechoslovakia and his occupation was "flipping" houses—buying houses, restoring or improving them, and then reselling them. George had the aristocratic manners of old Europe and the financial know-how of the flintiest businessman. He and his partner, Lloyd Burr, lived in the Hollywood Hills.

Besides being a patient, George and his partner Lloyd soon became good friends with Jack and me, dining at their house on several occasions. When Jack and I moved to Valley Village, George had loaned me money to help buy our condo. My Midwestern values were such that I borrowed from no one other than the bank and George. (It was only later I learned that hefty down payments on California real estate were misguided when the value of one's property could easily zero out with fire or earthquakes, as mine did after the Northridge earthquake of 1994.) In any case, one of my most haunting memories is that of sitting down to dinner at George and Lloyd's, with Jack and me on one side of the table, George and Lloyd across from us, eating a modest dinner. Anticipatory grief is missing someone while they're still alive and I was missing every one of these three already. Does anticipatory grief apply to missing a gathering, an event, while it is still ongoing? I think so. I tried, even then, to freeze such images in my mind as I was acutely aware we were all living on borrowed time and that such pleasant events could not last. We were, after all, the children of Hamelin and my sense of foreboding was all too accurate. Of the group, Jack would be the first to die. Later, Lloyd's alcoholism led to his own violent death in that very dining room and George, the last of the three, wouldn't survive the ravages of "Compound Q." And yet there stands that image of our group enjoying the simplest of pleasures and camaraderie—making an everyday salad, sitting down together for dinner—as if we were shielded from the bombs exploding around us and had all the time in the world. It is a memory that comes back to me time and again for I am successful in preserving those images, but am painfully aware that I am the only one left to recall them.

FRED LAWRENCE'S EX-WIFE
TRUST

Early on at LMG, on the chart placed on the door of the examination room, I found a female patient's name. Placing the patient's chart outside the exam room is a foundation of clinical practice for obvious reasons and is unlikely to change. In any case, I found this chart without the routine polaroid photo attachment. According to her file, she appeared very healthy and was HIV-negative. Half prepared, I adjusted myself for a new patient, at least new to me.

She was Fred Lawrence's ex-wife, in for her annual physical. At first I wondered why she was given to me. Ignoring the riddle, I provided her with one of the best exams I've ever performed. The write-up afterwards was similarly one of the better ones of my career. (I've read the post-mortem of President John F. Kennedy and I've questioned why it seemed to have been performed by a first-year medical student.) Although one is never to treat their own family, I never asked why Fred had given a VIP patient to me in particular.

As my time at LMG progressed, I also did exams of Fred's mother who was our Chief Financial Officer, as well as Fred's brother and his nephew. I understood the responsibility for these exams was a testament to Fred's faith in me.

THE WORST MOMENT

Learning of their HIV status was usually the very worst moment of someone's life. Like my own experience in San Francisco, the office employed the only reasonable policy: we never gave results, positive or negative, over the telephone and it was best to have our psychologist available. Without this policy clearly stated in advance, asking someone to come in for an office visit would have telegraphed their status. But once the individual was in the exam room, I would present the report, convey a certainty about the finding, but also provide some of that ingredient which keeps us all alive—hope.

Giving an HIV result was an excruciating part of the practice. The finding had to be given immediately. This is an obvious practice that applies to any discrete, black-or-white test. I only mention it here for those who may not be knowledgeable about standard medical practice. Whether or not I knew the patient, whether or not I had managed to establish a rapport when they had first come in for the test, the individual had to be told the test result immediately. It was not my place to judge the psychological strength of the man sitting in front of me. It would have been horribly condescending to delay giving the result for any reason.

Before breaking the news, not just of an HIV result but also of other non-emergency diagnoses, I would take a minute in the hallway to still myself—to separate from whatever I had been dealing with before. After having told the staff that I could not take calls, I would walk into the room and sit down. When a physician stands, it gives a message that he is in a hurry and on his way out; it gives the impression that the patient doesn't have his undivided attention or, worse, that the issue at hand is considered inconsequential. Whoever was receiving this information deserved his doctor's full attention and eye-to-eye intimacy. There would be no beating around the bush or drama as I would tell the patient immediately in no uncertain terms. There could be no confusion that either the test had been performed incorrectly or that the result might be that of someone else. I'd answer their questions of "Are you sure it's positive? Are you sure this is my test?" There was no mistake here: the results were what they were and without a doubt applied to the person sitting in front of me.

After the certainty of the test results, I'd present the uncertainty of prognosis—which was, after all, a piece of hope. I would give them the truth about epidemics in general. Carefully avoiding the word "survive" and instead favoring the softer expression "do well," I'd say yes, this was a bad finding, but in every epidemic throughout history there were those who did well. In HIV we didn't know who these people were, but that was cause for hope. At that time we had no other indicators of HIV progression such as "viral burden" which is a measurement of viral particles in the blood, nor did we know of the natural resistance of those missing the CCR5 gene. At that time we only had HIV status and T4 counts. And while AZT had been approved in 1987, even if a patient could tolerate the side-effects, frequently the gradual drift downward of a patient's white blood cell count forced discontinuation. Although AZT could usually buy a little time, clearly it was a blunt instrument. (When I would draw a bead, in fantasy, on our lethal target I was always unimpressed with its simple entity as a package of two nanoscopic twins of genetic encoding.) The great advances in anti-HIV medications weren't to appear until the mid-1990s. Therefore, even when pressed by a patient or his family, I did my best to avoid estimates of any one particular person's lifespan—my non-scientific, anecdotal observations of what appeared to me to be a 10% long-term survival rate was absolutely unfounded. It wasn't for me to blindly guess someone's chances of accelerated worsening or extended survival.

As part of this strategy, I wouldn't answer questions which weren't asked; I would wait for the patient to lead me to their hopes and fears. I wouldn't rush. I would take my time.

But every time I would give a little hope, a voice would whisper in my ear: "but not for you." The odds for any of us weren't good: even should the long-term survival rate be 30%, the mortality rate would still stand at a catastrophic 70%. (Dr. Paul Volberding, a famous early researcher, now estimates that, without therapy, long-term survival is less than 3%.)

Thus the pivotal statistics of survival, mortality, therapeutic effectiveness, etc. were not yet fully determined. Without this kind of numeric information, however, words became of greater consequence. As physicians our education and training had been steeped in numbers—from measurements of fasting blood sugars to ventilator oxygen limits to artery blockage fractions and, indeed, percentages of survival for various diseases. But our intellectual agility was tested in this new world of HIV in which the importance of metrics began to recede. Greg Pauxtis, M.D., an early HIV neurologist, has observed that those of us who were practicing at the time experienced a gradual revolution in our thinking—we began to reason not so much in numbers as in words. Our preoccupation with calculations drifted away and our discussions became dominated by words—words like "help" and "care" and "concern." The vital phrases of support, encouragement and affection that migrated into our thoughts and conversations had very little to do with mathematics.

So I believed I was not to survive this virus. And, odds were, neither were my patients. So it was with much amazement that I gradually came to realize that I was one of those fortunate few who were to survive years—if not many years. It was bittersweet irony when it became clear that I would live to see most of my patients die.

GIVING THE NEWS

Besides giving an HIV test result, an excruciating part of the practice was informing a patient that they would soon die. A person could be desperately sick in a hospital bed and yet be in complete denial. For others, their inexperience with the disease could sometimes lead to an ignorance of not only HIV's progression, but also the form of the illness which was soon to take their life. In either case, there could be great benefit for the patient in knowing their immediate future. They could inform their loved ones who could provide support or presence. They could provide instruction for their after-death affairs. But at this point there was not usually time for them to make peace with someone, write a will, or do other tasks. And there were others, like my own Jack, who couldn't tolerate the news—but, regardless, they needed to be told. There were also the moments when it was unclear even to me how close they were to death. This judgment, the right call, not the "if" but the "how" of telling patients my own estimate of the desperate seriousness of their illness was just as much a part of my practice as ordering tests and writing prescriptions.

Yes, some were ready; they had determined that their symptoms crescendoed in death. Others were in such denial that even increasing symptoms didn't penetrate their consciousness. It was my duty, my solemn work, to not only surmise the seriousness of their disease but also to map this terrain of the soul and convey the gravity of the situation while not leaving any room for misunderstanding or confusion. Or, in these particular situations, to not give any suggestion that would lead to false hope.

We must be honest with ourselves and our patients. We can't "do everything" and "save everyone." To ask someone how far they

ANDREW M. FAULK, M.D.

would want us to go in the attempt to preserve their life is profoundly difficult. The most important piece of information which needs to be conveyed is the probability of success. It is not easy to inform someone that, if their heart were to stop and their breathing cease, it is doubtful they would survive our efforts to retrieve them, and even if our efforts were successful, how long would they live afterward? We must be truthful in telling someone with end-stage AIDS that their life following resuscitation would usually be short in time and tormented in health. Also few people know of the force which is used in attempting to reverse the event: an attending once told me that CPR isn't administered correctly unless ribs are broken. This is hyperbole, but the concept is hard to miss. The truth must be told that suffering will be prolonged and for what purpose? Death is at hand whether we're successful in giving them a few more hours or not. Resuscitation doesn't change the ultimate course of their disease; we must be clear in providing an accurate prognosis.

Even if not in immediate danger, it is always best to discuss Code status before there is need. But the discussion is so much more difficult if the decision needs to be made quickly. If a Code is called and a DNR (Do Not Resuscitate) is not in effect, a hospital's machinery fully engages; it cannot be stopped. There can be no question, no deliberation, no calling of loved ones or assessment of probable success. Should someone be in the room at that moment and object to a resuscitation attempt, a Code cannot be aborted. There may be factors, after all, of which the Code team is unaware. Is the person protesting the resuscitation the responsible party? Do they have medical power of attorney? Would it be in this person's best interest for the patient to die? Are there inheritance issues? No, Code status was a decision that had to be worked out in advance, in thoughtful, unhurried moments.

Unless communication with the patient was absolutely impossible, it is always his or her choice. In order to make such a determination, of course, the patient needs to be as informed as possible. Discussing Code status is emotionally charged for both patient and physician. I don't mean to minimize the magnitude of difference in receiving this news versus giving it; even as a physician, or perhaps because I am a physician, I imagine how difficult it is for someone to grasp the gravity of the decision. To begin to hold this discussion is grueling. For me, and no doubt for any physician, it is always a schizophrenic moment. The human in me wants the patient to survive; the doctor in me knows this is an impossibility. Even though this could be excruciating in my exam rooms, these moments in the hospital, on the other hand, seemed to require the impossible: to present hope and reality in equal parts.

Years later, my own physician, Mark Higgins, M.D., emphasized that a person's all-important expectations depended on how many people with AIDS he knew, because this experience provided insight words couldn't. Many patients who had watched their counts drift lower and lower knew others who had preceded them and were ready, or at least knowledgeable. I will never forget those who had the gallows humor to joke about naming each of their few remaining T-cells. I found that those who were most ready for the worst news, not surprisingly, were those who had begun experiencing that long list of "take-aways" that HIV demanded—those who had lost their friends and faculties, their capabilities and independence, those who had had illness after illness until the disease simply wore them out. There were those who had been scorched by the fire and were ready to step off the earth.

* * *

One of the most memorable patients was a man in his early thirties who presented in the office without having had previous medical care. At 6' he probably weighed no more than 160 lbs.; one could see that he had once been remarkably handsome. Light blue eyes with jet black hair, perhaps "Black Irish," he worked as a sales clerk in a local high-end department store. Besides the obvious weight loss, his face was marked by the telling seborrheic dermatitis with its heavy flaking and redness at the edges of his nose and the space between his eyebrows. In his case, the staff had taken one look at him, listened to his complaints and sent him for a chest X-ray even before I had seen him. I did a quick exam, listened to his lungs and then took his film into the hall where our light box was located. His chest X-ray was a deadly blanket of *Pneumocystis* snow.

I walked back into the exam room and told him it looked like a bad pneumonia and he would need to be admitted to the hospital immediately. "I've never had a sick day in my life," he volunteered. I looked into his eyes; not only did he almost certainly have PCP, but his HIV was advanced and the length of his life could probably be measured in days, maybe weeks, but certainly not months.

I didn't tell him that he had PCP, that he had AIDS. Those had been critical minutes in that exam room. I had been responsible for conveying my assessment, but I had resisted giving him the truth, the almost certain truth.

After that patient left for the hospital, Fred took me aside. He had overheard my parting comments in the hall and had surmised what had occurred. In his role as an "old hand" at AIDS in those horrific years, he was troubled by what I had told the once beautiful man that had just left my exam room, or rather by what I hadn't said. I had been wrong, Fred told me, I should have told him the obvious truth that he had AIDS.

Although this patient's chest X-ray was consistent with PCP, an unequivocal diagnosis couldn't be made from that alone. His laboratory data hadn't yet been determined. To inform the patient, was *absolute* certainty required? Or was our considerable experience sufficient for gut-wrenching pronouncement?

But Fred had seen another factor at play that I hadn't seen myself. Fred had detected my subconscious wish that the news not be true—a yearning for the man standing before me not to be doomed. Although the patient's specific data wasn't yet known, should he have been told the journey to his death had begun? Did I not tell him because I didn't want to believe it? Had I allowed my own emotions to come first?

I hadn't told him he had AIDS. On which motivation had my action been based?

How and when to give the news was a vital part of our practice. But I believed that telling him, telling anyone, depended on the completeness of objective findings. In the end I hadn't told him, not because of my emotions, but because our findings were incomplete. It was a weighty reminder, however, that what I wished for could not influence my work.

LUKE OLSON, M.D.
THE WORLD CRASHING DOWN

It is difficult to convey the sense of the world crashing down around us in those years of the late 1980s and early 1990s. Our staff was as susceptible to infection as our patients and we worked in an unsteady atmosphere of constant loss. Lawrence Medical rarely terminated office and medical assistants, but it wasn't uncommon for employees to leave the practice due to the emotionally overwhelming nature of our work. Unexpected losses were particularly disturbing—we were, after all, under siege and each disappearance was keenly felt. In spite of this environment, it was with surprise and consternation we learned one day that one of our assistants had been found dead in his car on a shoulder of Interstate 405—a suicide unforeseen by our staff. I had barely known him.

Vincent was a gregarious man and so it was common to be meeting his new acquaintances. Two sports medicine physicians that he introduced to me were Tom and Stephen, who were robust body builders. They had been partners outside the office but in spite of their separation their deprecating humor revealed their continuing affection for each other. They were especially engaging and, upon meeting them, Tom invited me and my Significant Other to his birthday party the following Saturday. Jack and I attended the event held at Tom's house in the Olympus subdivision of the city which, besides stunning views of the valleys below, had a large deck perfect for the party. The get-together was an elaborate affair with over 30 guests and both doctors dramatically wearing only white. The hors d'oeuvres were delicious and the toasts heartfelt.

But I rarely referred a patient for a sports medicine consult and as a result I didn't interact with the two. It was a full six months later when I asked Vincent if he was seeing much of them. In spite of our work I was still surprised by Vincent's response: Stephen had succumbed three months after I met him and Tom had died the previous week. Vincent would be attending his funeral.

These were also times of grotesque irony. Phil and John weren't lovers, only room-mates, and were both seen by me. John, the older of the two, was a hypochondriac who did, at last, come into the office with a quarter-sized KS lesion on his neck. They had lived in hope they would never hear the bad news, but nevertheless feared it was in their future and that the unfortunate day had indeed arrived. Before John's KS lesion, his hypochondria had made him the focus of their joint attention which only skyrocketed after his diagnosis. His mother flew in from Philadelphia and we had multiple family conferences involving her, a brother in town and, of course, Phil. For a time I was receiving daily calls from either John or Phil concerning John's illness.

Six weeks after John's diagnosis, Phil called with fevers and a bad cough. I told him to meet me in the ER and there I discovered that his chest X-ray was "whited out." We started therapy immediately and, while he initially responded, he nevertheless died within a month. John, on the other hand, survived for another year. It was an era of ironies.

In the last few months of 1990 the world truly seemed to be falling apart, when I was asked to care for one of our own docs from the office. While staff deaths were deeply disconcerting, we had never had one of our own physicians sicken. Luke Olson, M.D., had always looked gaunt in the way HIV produces; he had the hallmark emaciation with prominent facial wasting and bi-temporal fat loss. Additionally, I had heard that Luke was "extraordinarily strange" from a staff member with whom he shared an apartment; however, I was to discover soon enough that it was something more than mere eccentricity.

Before I saw him, Luke's condition had put him in the hospital where I was to interview and examine him. The door to his room had the usual patient's name with his attending physician's name beneath it. As I brushed past the door, did I see "Olson/Dr. Faulk" or did I see "Faulk/Dr. Olson"? As I walked in the room, Luke was sitting up in bed with his hospital gown sagging with one side half undone. He was embarrassed—embarrassed to be hospitalized, embarrassed to be in a hospital gown, embarrassed to be in front of me. Embarrassed to be sick.

As I walked into the room, Luke sat with sunken temples and concave cheeks, sweating in a cold room, sipping water from a white styrofoam cup. I saw myself in that bed: gaunt, forlorn, needlessly ashamed. Here I was, examining a physician who had been my colleague only days before. As I sat down next to his bed, a new patient was rolled in to share his room, which annoyed and distracted me. Many times Luke and I had sat across from each other in the LMG doctors' lounge, each working silently on our separate patient's charting. Here, with the chatter of nurses and patients banging around us, in the midst of one of the most sensitive conversations of our lives, we had neither quiet nor privacy.

He had been a professional confidant. Was I taking his medical history or was he taking mine?

Both of us felt awkward but it wasn't long before the details of his self-treatment spilled out of him like a penitent confessing to his priest. His diet had been strikingly different from the one he had been recommending to his patients only days before. He had been a vegetarian for how many months he couldn't remember. While I am not educated in vegetarian diets, I can speak from experience: in a disease known for its malnutrition, vegetarian diets were almost always associated with precipitous deaths. Not that this was the only difficulty, necessarily, but I question the absorption of iron in AIDS. Iron is complexed in red meat in such a way that absorption occurs more readily than in vegetables and this seemed to be particularly relevant in my patients. But Luke's reason for excluding meat from his diet was one I had not heard before: he didn't eat meat because it made his urine taste particularly disagreeable. In some East Indian tradition, Luke had been drinking his own urine. Refrigeration, he also explained, made his urine more palatable. I could not imagine the consternation which our office assistant must have experienced when he first stumbled upon a container of urine cooling in his refrigerator.

My face remained expressionless. With people healthy one day and dead the next, disconnected families worrying about appearances, patients dying before their families even knew they were gay, people falling off radar only to be found dead next to busy freeways—all in a narcissistic society distant and apathetic. I was still surprised by Luke's admission. But whatever choices he'd made, I sat there without condemnation. Who was I to judge what paths someone took in attempt to escape the hangman's noose? In order to avoid some freak infection, Norman Nash hadn't simply rinsed his produce, his apples, oranges and peaches, he had diligently scrubbed them with soap and water. Luke had tried an unconventional, even bizarre, route to escape the juggernaut fast on his heels. Would some future doctor, safe in his or her world, sit in judgment of whatever decisions he had made? Perhaps the best personal maneuver, in the face of research that hadn't yet found treatment or cure, was to try various remedies, no matter how extraordinary or unlikely. The Scientific Method would eventually wend its way to a conclusion, but the quick return might be an answer of silence. Instead of waiting for charts—statistics—studies—algorithms—numbers—diagrams, he had chosen to act. His particular choice had proven dreadfully misguided; in HIV, depending on one's own urine for protein was tantamount to suicide. But what if his particular decision had been effective? I was waiting for scientific answers; he had not.

I watched as Luke, my co-worker, quickly succumbed in the following days. Between his inadequate diet and the ingestion of urine, he was extraordinarily malnourished which hastened his death. I felt that I didn't have the time, or psychological energy, to mourn his death as I thought I would have in a world less pressed with loss. The full expression of grief was a luxury I thought none of us had; emotional withdrawal seemed the only option. But Luke's passing pricked my professional detachment and drew blood.

AS WE RUN INTO THE FIRE

It is difficult to describe the events of that period, to convey the crushing deluge of this terrible time. By the end of 1987 over 47,000 people had died in the United States[2], hollowing out the gay communities of every major city before our eyes (approx. 58,000 Americans died in the Vietnam War). Dr. Paul Volberding tells medical students today that AIDS was more remote than polio when he started his training: "It's important to remember how devastating and stigmatizing this disease was." To the world the crisis may have been invisible, but to us it was a war zone we lived in from which there was no respite. For me to endure, I thought, the horrible weight had to be managed, compartmentalized; I needed to shut down my emotions. But it is the nature of the human psyche and the times that these walls of protection proved permeable at unexpected times.

One staff assistant, Carlos, had been a practicing physician in a Central American country, but was not licensed in the US. He was a quiet man, but not because of any language barrier since his English was excellent. It was his job to take a patient's vital signs (temperature, weight, etc.) and usher patients in and out of exam rooms, so I was a little confused one day to find him remaining in a room with a patient, Michael—a man who had obviously been exceptionally handsome before HIV's assault, but now so thin that he looked as though shaking his hand would crack a bone. Even with the physical and psychological exhaustion that accompanies caring for someone with a terminal illness, Michael had become Carlos' lover.

But Michael's decline couldn't be stopped and we watched sadly as they fearlessly faced the end and moved in together. They only had a couple of months before he died, but in this instance unexpected cracks in my emotional barricades allowed me to grieve with Carlos.

Looking back years later, I didn't discuss my emotional detachment with anyone as I calculated that the full expression of grief was a luxury I couldn't afford; I shut down emotionally to protect that core of me that could still feel something. It is clear to me now that a trained psychologist would've been of great help, but I was blind to the possibility that this would have had meaningful impact. The citizens of America conducted business as usual; the world outside our confines seemed untroubled and unaffected. Instead of daily body counts, our countrymen watched *Cheers* and *The Golden Girls*. I was busy beyond words and yet I wasn't able to keep people from the edge, they were slipping off the earth and I feared I was only giving them companionship along the way. I'd drive home, exhausted after a day of seeing patients, signing death certificates and taking calls from frantic patients or their families terrified about a lesion or desperate for information about possible new treatment developments. Sometimes when I'd be washing my chapped hands in some hospital room sink, I'd absent-mindedly ponder how someone my age should be out enjoying life instead of inside, writing orders for men I knew wouldn't live. We were the ones running into the fire, into the burning house, while others were running away from the flames—escaping to Palm Springs, to Bucks County, to Guerneville, or into mind-numbing jobs or unfulfilling relationships—escaping the deluge of loss and grief and the burden of caring for those for whom it was too late to flee and from whom there was the horrific possibility of contracting the disease.

In society's neglect and opprobrium, the government's budget for HIV research was always absurdly small compared to the number of people dying. Too often families participated in this cover-up by hiding the deaths of their loved ones behind the words "pneumonia" and "cancer." On more than one occasion a brother or sister would plead with me not to disclose the reason for death to a parent, but ACT UP's war cry was bitter truth: "Silence Equals Death" and the accuracy of HIV statistics was too important to muddy. I always told legal next-of-kin what I documented on death certificates; what was told to friends and relatives outside of these interactions was obviously out of my control.

Politically, some of the first questions concerning AIDS arose at a White House press briefing in October of 1982. The response of President Ronald Reagan's Deputy Press Secretary, Larry Speakes, was stomach-churning, homophobic lightheartedness, which was met with unconcealed laughter by press pool reporters. For several years after this, questions in other White House press briefings were made, and answered, with the same sickening jocularity. The nauseating "humor" in these give-and-take interchanges revolved around gay-bashing questions about reporters' sexual orientation. These exchanges and government inaction were based on the fact that the epidemic was largely confined to the gay community. Had the general population been subject to infection and death, these rejoinders would have been viewed as callous and inhumane, as they were. Obviously these responses were not limited to public relations; this was the attitude of the government at large and, indeed, society.

Through most of his years in office, Reagan quarreled with his Surgeon General, C. Everett Koop, about whether AIDS should be medically addressed, let alone publicly acknowledged. Reagan's lack of leadership, if not outright obstruction, was deadly: it rationalized minuscule research funding and fueled mainstream fear and hatred of gay men. Consider that Mayor Dianne Feinstein's AIDS budget for the City of San Francisco was bigger than President Reagan's AIDS budget for the entire nation for two years in a row in the mid-80s. The President's pointed funding resistance reinforced the hostile zealotry of Christian Evangelicals, such as Baptist minister Jerry Falwell, Sr., a co-founder of the Moral Majority, who preached that "AIDS was the wrath of God on homosexuals," and "AIDS is not just God's punishment for homosexuals. It's God's punishment for the society that tolerates homosexuals." At one point, late in his presidency, Reagan said "When it comes to preventing AIDS, don't medicine and morality teach the same lessons?" The nation's Catholic cardinals, predictably, preached against gay rights as Reagan's Communications Director, Pat Buchanan, stated that AIDS was "nature's revenge on gay men."

Thus the epidemic was compounded by a society which left us and our dying brothers largely abandoned and, initially, without services from kitchens to mortuaries. To their great credit it was the lesbian community, as well as many heterosexual groups, that jumped in to orchestrate AIDS fundraising and education. Pockets of Catholic charities (after their rejection of papal sensibilities) were known for giving one-on-one care—a mark of true dedication and self-sacrifice. They were the groups who, led by their sense of active compassion, began and staffed hospices, ran food delivery services to the house-bound and held the hand of the dying when their families shunned them. AIDS was catastrophic for the gay community and its supporters, but it frequently minimized our differences and bettered the world of the sick and the poor.

ACT UP

It was ACT UP (AIDS Coalition to Unleash Power), begun in 1987 and lasting a decade, that saw the death surrounding us and demanded society see the same. ACT UP was a welcome, and absolutely essential, force in publicizing the inadequate resources devoted to HIV research and treatment. In the war against AIDS, battles were being fought at the bedsides of patients, in the halls of hospitals, in anxious family waiting rooms, and in government research centers and pharmaceutical boardrooms. We also struggled with the media to change its recalcitrant policies and inform the public about the societal discrimination and indifference we faced. In fact it was institutional neglect from many different sources that drove the pioneers of ACT UP to organize resistance and develop their own brand of societal activism.

Against seemingly intractable power, with no more than 10,000 activists, ACT UP fought for basic change. Larry Kramer (1935-2020), author of *The Normal Heart*, was one of the founders of the Gay Men's Health Crisis that morphed into ACT UP. In these words he distilled their goals and overarching approach: "I was trying to make people united and angry. I was known as the angriest man in the world, mainly because I discovered that anger got you further than being nice."

Coalescing gay men and recruiting devoted lesbians, ACT UP was a tremendous force in pressuring the FDA to release drugs expeditiously and have them priced reasonably; indeed, when AZT was first approved it was the most expensive medication in the US. "Silence=Death," their haunting logo, was genius in its truth, as was their use of the pink triangle (the Nazis used the pink triangle point-down to identify gay people and, when superimposed on a yellow Star of David, simultaneously identified one as both homosexual and Jewish). "United in anger!" was their battle cry as they threw ferocious urgency into the fight to revolutionize the priorities of the government and pharmaceutical companies. As our brothers were dying all around us, ACT UP demanded to know how those unaffected could continue on without any interruption in their lives.

While I faced the government's indifferent and meager responses every day in the clinic and hospital, the hours I was working and the time I needed to monitor journals and decompress at home tended to insulate me from the news. However I knew of their overnight sleep-ins and vigils in early 1988 and 1989 in the L.A. County/USC hospital in order to establish a dedicated AIDS unit there. My heart was with ACT UP, but my place wasn't chained to truck axles and hand-cuffed to pharmaceutical company gates. Instead I focused on the care and medical advocacy for each of my patients which frequently involved being on the phone with insurance companies for 20 minutes or longer. HIV was new, of course, and the companies were mystified by our various medications and methods, but whether people were dying or not, they searched for reasons to disapprove necessary funding. Just as today the pharmaceutical companies fought for their 22% profit.

I attended the San Francisco International AIDS Conference in June of 1990, on behalf of LMG, in order to present the latest findings to our group and the L.A. community. Upon walking back to the Moscone Center one day after lunch, my colleagues and I, our name tags clearly identifying us as assembly participants, were pelted by water balloons thrown by ACT UP members. As attendees, we were some of those most dedicated to funding AIDS research and treatment as well as expediting drug release and affordability; obviously to bombard us with water balloons was painfully misguided. For quite some time my impression of ACT UP was conflicted. No doubt influenced by this unfortunate event and what little I heard in the national news, I believed their efforts involved indiscriminate targeting of the general public and the medical community.

Even though it was a mistake to test their pitching accuracy on us, ACT UP understood the significance of the government disregard for that important international conference. The 1987 ban on HIV-infected people entering the US hobbled the assembly as foreign scientists, including the important French co-founders of the virus, boycotted the event in solidarity with HIV-positive researchers and patients. Similarly blocking traffic on the Golden Gate Bridge during rush hour in January, 1989, may have appeared to be the right thing to do in making our fellow citizens aware of our mounting losses, but San Franciscans were at the forefront of AIDS efforts and I felt worsening traffic snarls for them gained us neither favor nor progress. I knew these incidents, however, were just minor collateral damage from the aggressive actions that were imperative and I concede that it was better to do too much rather than too little. The system—the government, the insurance companies, the drug companies—all failed us in many more ways than just erecting bureaucratic hoops and impediments. Their apathy and greed were bleeding the gay community. Silence was death.

IN THE MIDST OF WAR

At Lawrence Medical, for some time I served on call every third week and weekend. The on-call physician covered hospitalized patients with their great demand for consultation with specialists, families and significant others. It was a testament to Fred Lawrence's dedication and hands-on mindset that he himself was performing the same amount of on-call coverage as Vincent and I. With the epidemic, Lawrence Medical had experienced an explosion of cases; Vincent and Fred's workloads had skyrocketed before I joined the practice. They had worked tirelessly during the initial burst of AIDS as the practice grew exponentially. Although AZT had been approved by the FDA in 1987, its efficacy seemed spotty and many patients couldn't tolerate the side-effects. I questioned whether it actually extended life in those with less than 200 T-cells. The growth of hours and our availability was good for the budget but there also was a deep sense, shared by the entire office, that we were doing something of profound importance. We were functioning in a plague, in the midst of a war. Most doctors of the time either didn't want the extra work in treating HIV or weren't sure how. On the other end of the spectrum were the purveyors of nonsense.

The years I was in practice I had built a body of knowledge and experience that forswore the chasing of one medication or therapy after another. Especially in the early years of the epidemic, urgency and ignorance produced a wild rush for anything that offered a gleam of hope and what I saw was sometimes improvement but, more often than not, disease acceleration. This provoked a profound skepticism in me about using untried medications. Although there was always the chance we were missing out on some new effective treatment, unless it was part of a study, I came to believe there was no point in becoming crazy by chasing rumors.

We would hear of doctors who were practicing suboptimal medicine. And there were reports, backed by evidence, of some few M.D.s practicing a type of medicine which at best showed incredibly poor judgment and at worst was a particularly vicious form of fraud. The most questionable practitioners would treat their patients with Chinese herbs, acupuncture, Dale Carnegie positive thinking, Louise Hay visualization, camaraderie (e.g., "Hay rides") and various nutrient-challenged diets. Then there were the "practitioners" who opted for various therapies based on "imbalances," methods of consumption, diet, mold or meditation alone. These charlatans and self-deceivers would "treat" these patients, my brothers, until their condition was grave and then, in order to be able to report glowing statistics of homeopathic success, transfer them to us soon before they died for conventional care by legitimate physicians.

Perhaps I spend too much effort on my polemic against these people, but their destructive ignorance and magical thinking surrounded us and gave us at LMG another mission, a special mission. After presenting patients of these practitioners with the news of being HIV-positive or having an opportunistic infection, I would spend considerable time explaining that their lack of a positive attitude or visualizations were not to blame. You have a bad disease, I would repeat over and over, you are not responsible for all of this. With these kinds of pressures, it was easy to see we had a special calling. Physicians have special obligations in times of crisis: I, for one, was running into the burning house.

LOUISE HAY
GUILT

Louise Hay was everywhere at the time. I never heard her speak, I never read a book she wrote, yet I dealt with her every day in my office. It may have been the EST movement which first started promoting the concept that people are responsible for everything that happens to them. But what I constantly saw in my office was the belief system of Louise Hay which evidently taught that those who are ill are ultimately responsible for their own illness. When I saw Tom, or Ed, or Bill in the exam room, almost to a man they felt both sick and guilty. While I am not by any means an authority on her various beliefs and practices, I saw the aftermath of her work, for what she taught landed front and center in those exam rooms on Wilshire Boulevard. One might imagine that, if there were fault, it was from whatever indiscretion had left my patients with the infection in the first place. No, that wasn't the guilt I dealt with every day in my office. My patients were struggling with the suffocating responsibility expressed in the ideas of Hay and her disciples.

Hay was born in 1926 and divined from a diagnosis of cervical cancer in 1977 or '78 that positive thinking could heal the body. She believed that forgiveness, therapy, nutrition, reflexology, and enemas were the route to healing; she authored several self-help books, the most influential being the 1984 book entitled *You Can Heal Your Life* ("If you can change your thinking you can change your life"). According to Louise Hay, in promoting this vision, she was the voice of a prophet in a sick and suffering world. That same year she began leading support groups in L.A. for people living with HIV which she called "Hay Rides." Those events grew from a few men in her living room to a large hall in West Hollywood. In March 1988, she appeared on both *The Oprah Winfrey Show* and *Donahue*.

How one views the various circumstances of life and how one constructs his life fundamentally affects his happiness and happiness, I believe, increases lifespan. Placebo and prayer, interestingly enough, have been shown to have an effect in fighting many cancers and conditions. In gauging the efficacy of prayer, it doesn't seem to matter whether the one who's praying is the patient or not, or has any degree of faith or religious commitment. Obviously one's attitude influences how one perceives his or her health. In every scientific experiment researching the benefit of any medication or therapy, there's always a placebo; if the mind had no input into one's health, a placebo would be unnecessary.

Hay's New Age thinking may have given us insights into the value of affirmative thought, but the flip-side of this principle is a brutal insistence on personal accountability: if one can heal oneself, one can make oneself ill. If one says your thoughts impact health, I agree. If one says your thoughts define your health, I disagree. I would deal with the guilt—day after day, patient after patient—of those sitting in front of me who thought they were sick because they hadn't visualized good health with sufficient conviction or precision. They were ill because their imagery was incorrect or incomplete. A distraught patient, coughing, with a temperature of 103 degrees, and 110 pounds on a 6'1" frame, would "confess" that if only he had visualized properly he would not be in my office. If only he had believed enough. And some would draw the harsh conclusion from the extrapolation of Hay system logic that one is sick because they choose to be.

As I sat there, listening to the confessions of my misguided patients, I would silently curse the fatuous, sanctimonious teachings of the omnipresent Louise Hay. While dealing with the medical gravity of, say, *Pneumocystis* pneumonia or Kaposi's Sarcoma, again and again I would need to begin by convincing my patients that imagination and visualizations, incantations and amulets couldn't provide protection against the virus. I battled daily with this crisis of my time and tribe.

Perhaps I give Hay too much credit in circulating this destructive mind-set, she may have just noted Susan Sontag's observations. Sontag describes the effect of religion on the way we describe diseases and argues that over time, Christianity forced connections between disease and morality, blaming patients for his or her own sickness. She asks whether we should then consider every psychological problem as an illness and whether every illness, in turn, should be considered the result of a psychological problem. Sontag notes that if that's the case, then everyone who is sick has become ill on purpose because they secretly want to, and so deserve to be sick.

In assisting my brothers deal with death, I worked scrupulously to avoid religious or philosophical convictions, but here the wounds from their guilt were too damaging, the concepts too misguided. "You've got a bad disease," I would say, "you can't visualize it away; neither thinking nor belief can cure you." And then, judging by the response of the individual—particularly listening to their choice of words—I would jump into what we knew of scientific treatment for their symptoms and disease and their priorities to achieve a happy life.

ADVICE AND THE UNKNOWN

My patients frequently felt that they needed to become medically educated overnight in order to survive their disease. Studies have shown better outcomes and greater happiness when patients are intimately involved in their own care. Before the Iron Curtain fell, global suicide rates were highest in Eastern Europe and it is commonly thought that they were a result of the lack of personal liberty, lack of individual autonomy. Although my men knew that proactive people did better, almost to a person they were confronted by a body of knowledge completely outside their education or experience. These were blue-collar workers and professionals of every stripe, all suddenly overcome by a staggering mountain of information. While it is optimal to be involved in one's own medical care, this can often be confusing and overwhelming in a routine disease, let alone in the intricacies of a new, poorly-understood retrovirus. Yet the majority of people I saw took on this tremendous burden.

Despite the benefit which results from knowing a great deal about one's illness, I was less a fan of self-education than my peers; admittedly, my viewpoint was not, and is not, the accepted wisdom. I didn't discourage patients from studying their illness, but it seemed to me that the most accurate information at the time was weighted toward the negative, the truth. Formal articles and fact-based reporting were filled with unsuccessful maneuvers and the percentages of those who died. There is advantage in being involved in one's own care, there is good in facing truth head-on, but this approach isn't always best for everyone at all times.

"I know you want to understand your problem," I would say, "and that's great. But you're attempting to educate yourself overnight about a newly-discovered, complex and poorly understood virus. It took me 11 years to become a physician. You can't do the same thing in two weeks. You're asking too much of yourself. Find a doctor you trust, somebody you can be completely honest with—it might not be me and that's all right—but find the right doctor and relax in his or her care. And then stay up on HIV as much as you want. Or can."

In spite of the enormous difficulty of this undertaking, I was frequently awed by the command of the illness some "civilians" articulated. But this was a two-edged sword: a little knowledge is a dangerous thing. I've been at international AIDS conferences at which lay people have made extraordinarily perceptive suggestions and penetrating insights, but I've also heard remarks which showed little command of the scientific process and would've been incredibly destructive if acted upon.

Sometimes patients in this terribly painful initial period would ask about survival time. I would answer them that, during any plague in human history, a certain percentage of people would, as I would phrase it, "do well." It might be genetics, or self-care, or any number of factors, but there were always people that would "do okay" over the long-term, I'd say. There was a chance, I would always acknowledge, that this person standing in front of me might do well. (On occasion I argued the imaginative logic that if you're one of the 1% that survive, then, for you, it is 100%.)

But after this I would attempt to gently steer them towards the metaphysical. "For you, what is the most important thing in the world?" "What makes your life meaningful?" I would never say "bucket list," but I would ask what it was that they had always wanted to do, what they had always wanted to see, where they had always wanted to go.

Even though this was the message I gave my patients, I never included myself in the 10% survival rate I appeared to be seeing—a rate merely anecdotal and definitely not scientific. My motto, as was that of every doctor at LMG, was "Hope for the best. Plan for the worst." I didn't see myself living past 1993; it is the irony of my life that I have lived as long as I have. In 1993, I was certain I would step off the earth before 1995. And then in 1995 protease inhibitors came on the scene and changed everyone's arithmetic.

PROBLEM PATIENTS

Throughout my years of medical practice, I had a routine which was perhaps a bold-faced abuse of my position. Every year at Christmas I would discharge one patient from my practice. Of course this was done by legal procedure with registered notice and gave the individual ample time to locate another provider. It involved a number of registered letters with the recipient's signature required. A list of other acceptable doctors was always a nice touch, but not a requirement.

From my rogue's gallery of overly-demanding patients, there were those who were impossible to please, those who could only be satisfied with impossible sacrifices on my part. There is a relief, a tremendous relaxation, found in the recognition that you are human and cannot please everyone. Fred was not happy with this custom I had carried with me from the dysfunctional San Francisco practice, but he nevertheless allowed this tampering with the practice. He recognized the pressure of our work.

So who was I to discharge from my practice and my psyche? I had a small collection from which to choose. They fell into two clusters: the first, and by far the largest, were those whose passive-aggressive natures sabotaged my medical treatment and who loudly complained of my ineffectual management of their illnesses. The other smaller group consisted of those incapable of recognizing my time and limitations. These were the "worried well," a group pointed out to us in medical school. Their sin lay in their trivial and impatient complaints which I could not help but compare to the desperate condition of their HIV-infected brothers. (I once received a call at 4 a.m. from one of these patients requesting a sleeping pill.)

Those few patients who were HIV-free knew full well the disease of the majority of our patients. If they had been ignorant, their demands and complaints would have been easier to excuse, but they were oblivious to the anguish surrounding them which was, for me, exasperating. Had our modest fame not been known, a visit to our waiting room would have made our practice apparent. Connections are crippled by resentment and irritation; strain should be the last thing to influence doctor-patient interaction and usually it can be avoided. But when it develops, maybe it is time for someone to send a registered letter.

FRED LAWRENCE, M.D.
AIDS EXPERTISE

Before the epidemic, many gay physicians had slipped into only treating Sexually Transmitted Diseases (STD). It was, compared to other fields, remarkably uncomplicated. But once STD medicine morphed into HIV medicine and the epidemic began to monopolize our attention, many of these doctors retired. To his credit, Dr. Lawrence was one of those who had spent the time and energy to develop his expertise in treating the immunocompromised. He had learned it—as I had—from its beginnings, which was no small feat; as one doc told me with only a little hyperbole, "If you know HIV medicine, you know medicine."

Those patients who were also his long-standing friends certainly benefited from his command of HIV medicine. But as time progressed, he gradually began transferring many of those patients to the care of Vincent and me. Fred was fond of repeating his personal maxim: "You don't need to *be* the best doctor, you just need to *hire* them." It was a compliment which made me smile inwardly every time I heard it, and perhaps revealed some of his thinking about those patients he transferred.

One of Fred's personal friends transferred to Vincent's care was Jeff Lysaght. Jeff was an extraordinarily engaging man with a somewhat eccentric handlebar mustache and ready remarks which displayed not only an intellectual prowess but also a command of the gallows humor in which we all participated from time to time. While he fell into my care only once or twice, it was more than enough to recognize him and hear his pungent remarks when we met in the LMG hallway as he headed toward Vincent's exam room. Jeff, in addition to whatever day job he held, volunteered at the annual gay rodeo held in nearby Burbank and it was always a pleasure to run into him, with his oversized mustache and his oversized wit, selling lottery tickets.

Although we were all too familiar with random news at random times, I never became used to hearing of the mounting deaths. While Jack and I had missed Jeff at the previous rodeo and I had missed passing him in our halls, I hadn't asked about him as I didn't want to know if he had taken the walk. I didn't inquire of those I no longer saw. So it was with more than a little consternation that I heard of Jeff's death from Fred in that casual, unaffected manner of that time period. It seemed Jeff had succumbed to a pneumonia—perhaps PCP or some other bacteria or virus in which the immunocompetent among us swim with unconscious impunity.

"Jeff was always afraid of drowning," Fred told me, "I guess in the end that's how he died." Fred and I were in his Mercedes driving home from one of our monthly office meetings. These get-togethers were held in a variety of restaurants with the tab, of course, being picked up by the office. As a remnant of the frugality of my life during the years of training, this felt like a grand luxury. During that particular business meeting, I had ordered a cocktail. I had thought little of it, although the gathering was devoted to the running of the office. In Fred's car, however, before he gave me the news about Jeff, he reprimanded me for the drink. In the darkness, I felt myself blushing. It was one innocent drink, but in my ridiculously hyperactive conscience the failing was as large as a missed laboratory test result.

As I pushed that discomfort out of my mind, he told me the news about Jeff's pneumonia and death. As usual, however, when discussing the passing of any of his friends or patients, his tone of voice was one of detached, resigned acceptance. But after the news, I was shocked when his hand reached across the car's console to the passenger's side where I was sitting and grasped my hand. His left hand remained on the steering wheel as he held my hand with his right. He continued driving in his usual terrifyingly high speed which had earned him multiple tickets and traffic school classes (although I strongly suspected that he arranged for others to attend these mandatory driving classes in his stead). With a little reflection,

I considered that while I may have chosen a drink, Fred chose to drive like a bat out of hell.

That night he held my hand in the car for what seemed like an eternity. Maybe it was an eternity. In spite of the emotional proximity with which I treated my patients, I was uncomfortable. I was ashamed of my discomfort, but then again, I was sitting in my boss' car as he held my hand. Soon enough, I saw how the extreme, the terrible, nature of our work had broken his heart. I relaxed. The world was upside-down—nothing was normal, nothing was abnormal.

MY SIGNATURE

During my first years in San Francisco in the 1980s, I attended a going-away party for a tall, thin man who was obviously ill. He was a member of a gay social club in the city and, instead of remaining in San Francisco, had decided to spend his final days back where he grew up in central Pennsylvania. I was unaccustomed to such a send-off, with its crushing heaviness. But as the epidemic ground on, farewells became more sudden and heart-wrenching as the community became familiar with both the devastating course of the disease and the possibility of actively controlling the timing of one's own death.

During my time of practice in L.A., I attended the "Goodbye Parties" of three of my patients and one of an acquaintance, all of which were far more intimate and heartbreaking than the send-off I had attended during those earliest years of the epidemic. All three of my patients had had partners and many friends who had preceded them in death and who had shown them, by example, the unkind end which the disease could cause. I had long talks with each. Most patients who consider physician-assisted suicide do so out of fear of uncontrolled pain and dismantling of autonomy. While I could assure them they could expect scrupulous pain management from me, outside of a metaphysical discussion I couldn't address issues of loss of independence. When we deal with the loss of physical autonomy, can't we perhaps consider this a potential lesson in humility for ourselves and possible emotional growth for our loved ones and caregivers? Despite the strength or weakness in these arguments, each of them feared loss of control over their bodies and societal independence and remained firm in the decision to end their lives. Some people find suicide against their beliefs and therefore they insist it be outlawed: I wonder about the *emotional imagination* of such individuals. One of our political parties seems to carry the same deficit—unless an event or condition happens to them personally, they can't imagine how it might be for another. A famous right-wing senator was tremendously hostile to LGBTQ rights until his daughter came out to him. Then, suddenly, this gentleman became pro-gay; the knowledge of a lesbian in the family had to be a personal circumstance in order for him to have awareness or empathy. It is unacceptable, to me, to argue that such a fundamental choice about your body, about your life, shouldn't be your own. In keeping with accepted standards in those states and countries where physician-assisted suicide was legal, I sent each to a doctor outside of LMG to confirm that they had no more than six months to live, and also to an associate psychiatrist to rule out depression or dementia.

These four chose the time of their death before the disease chose it for them. They had decided to make the end of their life a celebration; two of them maxed out their credit cards renting expensive hotel suites, having a DJ, providing an open bar, and catering food. One was in the Hotel Sofitel in L.A., a venue not as plush as its cost. As disturbing as it was to attend any of these "parties," I felt it was my responsibility—it was my signature, after all, on the prescription. F. Scott Fitzgerald wrote in *The Great Gatsby*, "Let us learn to show our friendship for a man when he is alive and not after he is dead." Attending Goodbye Parties, as incredibly heart-breaking as they were, was truly showing friendship for a man "when he is alive."

The ability of someone to come to grips with his own impending death, I found, has little to do with his capabilities in other parts of his life. We are all mortal, so why is it such a surprise to face our end? Certainly I know first hand this conundrum. I can be enjoying some trivial pleasure when the razor blade of awareness draws blood. Just when I think I've come to grips with my own death, a small thought throws me back to where I started. There is a veritable onion of feelings: I peel off one fear only to find another. As I turn my head toward some little pleasure of life, my mortality can slap me in the face.

As with most all of my practice, I didn't discuss Goodbye Parties with Jack. I kept these emotions to myself and dealt with them alone.

Thomas "Jerry" Bingham usually came into my office with one of two friends, either Kurt or Jim. The lines on his face, together with his longish greying hair, identified him in my mind as an aging hippie. He often teased me about the formality of my white lab coat over a shirt and tie. During many of my years in medicine I tended to look younger than I was and so, in my campaign for credibility, traditional medical clothing seemed best. But once I realized that connectedness was at the heart of what I could give my patients, I removed my coat and tie and unbuttoned my shirt.

Unhappily Jerry had between 100 and 200 T-cells and his visits with me had us watching their relentless drift downward as the disease progressed. His manner was bright, however, and he had that rare motivation, insight, and grace with which some patients make the physician feel better, rather than vice versa. As his T-cells dropped below 200, I placed him on pentamidine, an antibiotic commonly used at the time to treat and protect against PCP, the AIDS-related pneumonia.

Lawrence Medical did not assume the care of those without private insurance of some kind. But if a patient lost their coverage while under our care, they were never discharged from our practice. "Once a patient, always a patient" was the motto of Lawrence Medical and it was a philosophy that met my own sensibilities and ethics. Truth be told, I'd have preferred a practice which took everyone regardless of their insurance status, but losing one's insurance was frequent and we ended up treating many patients *gratis*. No matter his insurance, Jerry's care with us was secure. Our finance department, however, let me know his non-Medicaid insurance had collapsed and, more importantly, he was running out of money for non-medical expenses, although they were working with him on acquiring funds from AIDS Project Los Angeles (APLA). At various visits Jerry and I discussed his situation with Kurt and Jim. Kurt had offered Jerry a place to stay, but Kurt's finances were equally dire. And Jim had space constraints of his own.

In spite of these impediments, Jerry didn't seem to be depressed— just running out of options that he found acceptable. Unfortunately, he was one of the many to have extensive facial KS lesions and with each office visit there were more. Our staff knew our patients like family, but sometimes facial KS would so swell and disfigure faces that people weren't recognizable from one clinic visit to the next.

(The only social activity some of them would engage in was going to the movies at night so no one would notice them.) Jerry began to envision a future similar to that of those he knew who had passed before him, a future bereft of those things which made him happy. Kurt was with him in my office when he proposed a doctor-assisted suicide. Not in those words, of course.

"Hey, Doc, can you give me something to make it all go away?" I answered, "We're giving you everything we can, Jerry." He said, "No, Dr. Faulk, I mean everything." My eyes shot a glance to Kurt. "What do you mean exactly, Jerry?"

"I've lived a lot of good years, and all the ones ahead look bad. There are more KS lesions all the time and I can't look at myself in a mirror; I'm too embarrassed to leave my house. Can't you give me something to make me go to sleep?"

"Jerry, do you know what you're asking? Maybe another visit with our psychiatrist, Dr. Samuels, will help."

"I'm not depressed, Doc. I just don't want to go down the path that Mark did." (Mark had been his partner who had died two years earlier.)

"Well, I want you to really think about this. Do me a favor and see if APLA can't provide a different living situation. And why not see Samuels again?"

"I've thought about it already, Dr. Faulk, and I just don't want any more appointments. I like Dr. Samuels but the meds I'm on aren't changing my mind. I'm not sad. I'm just tired and I don't like what I see ahead of me."

We discussed this over a period of a month, but I asked him to make another appointment to see me in two weeks. After Jerry left my office, I called Martin Baines, our financial department's whiz kid. He told me that he had already spoken to Jerry about a number of possibilities and APLA had offered him their social workers and other county options which Jerry hadn't pursued. Peter Samuels, our psychologist, confirmed that Jerry wasn't depressed, just facing a grim future.

The next time I saw Jerry, both Kurt and Jim were with him. They confirmed that Jerry didn't seem depressed—just running out of alternatives.

His time ahead looked as bleak to me as it did to him, but my role was to give him as much encouragement as I could. I asked him to make one more appointment with our consulting psychiatrist—but I wrote him out the script just the same. The piece of paper seemed too small for what it could do. As I handed it to Jerry, I repeated my standard line for this situation, "Jerry, whatever you do, don't take all the pills at once and chase it with a fifth of gin."

In less than a week I heard back from our psychiatrist and Martin. Their evaluations had not changed. Jerry wasn't clinically depressed and APLA had discovered several housing options. That same day, however, Jerry called me on the phone. As they disrupted my schedule, I rarely took non-emergency calls during my workday; either I returned calls after I had seen my last patient of the day or in the morning before I had seen my first. But I knew this was not a usual phone call; I quickly took Jerry's call.

"Andrew," Jerry said, addressing me for the first time by my given name, "Kurt, Jim and I are having a little going away party on Sunday and it'd mean a lot to me if you could come."

"Are you sure you want to do this, Jerry?" I felt a chill run down my back.

"Yeah, I don't want to see what I see in the mirror anymore. I'm at rest with things going like this."

As I worked in our office on Saturdays, Sunday was a day I was available. Unlike most other Goodbye Parties, Jerry's send-off was not a lavish, extravagant affair—he evidently had never been in a position to nurture credit cards. So instead of a costly hotel suite, Jerry had his send-off at home.

He lived in a small ranch house in the San Fernando Valley heavily shaded by trees and, unlike his neighbors, a yard off to the side. Jerry's bedroom opened directly onto this large side-yard and he had moved his mattress from a bed to the floor in front of the doorway. For the most part, he remained on the mattress, legs folded into a lotus position. His roommates had set up a folding table outside with jug-wine, a few bottles of different liquors, and blue and red plastic cups. Jerry stayed on the mattress with the door open to the others, as his few visitors, with plastic cups in their hands, drifted between the bedroom and the yard. It was a warm day in the valley but not as horrendously hot as was common and I was thankful for the trees. In the living room a cheap stereo played a collection of rock pieces from the late 1970s and early '80s. All the windows of the house were open, and the music could easily be heard throughout the house and yard. I recognized one other patient of mine in the little group that had formed around the table and greeted him, awkwardly, and talked with him a bit. Searching for a topic, my patient kidded another guest about a wedding ring on the fourth finger of his left hand. The target of his tease replied that it was his personal technique for distancing aggressive women who approached him. Although everyone attending knew the purpose of the get-together, Jerry had been diplomatically circumspect about where the prescription had come from. At one point, one of the strangers asked me if I had written it. I answered him that he would have to ask Jerry.

Someone had brought orange juice which one or two of the guests mixed with vodka; the jug-wine on the table contributed to a feeling of informality. There were five or six people there when I arrived and the number grew no bigger than ten.

About half of his guests, in sitting with Jerry, teared up but it was a period in my life in which I didn't cry (Jack had not yet died) and I was thankful that keeping a dry eye wasn't a struggle for me. There were few exchanges in the yard among this somber group. But there at the doorstep, the conversations with Jerry, more often than not, were of common remembrances of various shared events. Once again I was struck by the comforting power of connection— connection which I now saw as crucial to patient care.

Jerry appeared determined and at peace with what was going to conclude the day. "Thanks, Andrew, for making this get-together possible." In spite of his intent, I found his comment deeply disturbing. I would have been at peace had I made this decision for myself, but there it was, my name signed on Jerry's prescription. I had sworn the oath of physicians throughout history: *primum non nocere*—above all, do no harm. My oath was to do what was best for those who had entrusted me with their well-being. Was I doing the right thing? Was this doing ultimate harm rather than ultimate good?

Repeatedly I spoke to him about the pills he was about to take.

"Jerry, you can change your mind at any time," I said. "If you do, tell Kurt or Jim and we'll have you hospitalized right away. Depending on the timing, it's likely that we'll have a good chance of success."

I imagined myself in Jerry's place. Should he change his mind at any point, I didn't want him to feel trapped by inertia or embarrassment. He was not to die in panic, no matter how far the medications had progressed. "I'm only a phone call away," I emphasized. I knew I'd be spending the rest of the afternoon and evening next to my phone. I calmed myself—should it come to that, I'd be able to more or less control emergency intervention as I knew which drugs were involved.

"No, Dr. Faulk, that won't happen. I won't be needing your services any more." Jerry's return to formality reinforced my heavy responsibility. "But I thank you for all the help you've been to me. You were always there when I needed you. You're a good man."

I probably spent 30 minutes sitting on Jerry's doorway stoop while he reclined a few feet away on the mattress. Out in the yard Kurt and Jim quietly thanked me but their gratitude provoked mixed emotions. My prescription would kill my patient; handwriting on a piece of paper would end Jerry's life. My handwriting. My signature.

Finally I left the gathering—that little, modest accumulation of his closest friends and few possessions. If I were him, would I have chosen this clean break, this simple walk to the edge? Could I swallow all those pills knowing that they would carry me off the earth? To know the probable course of a disease isn't the same as knowing with certainty how it would evolve in a specific person. Neither Jerry nor I knew how AIDS might progress in his particular case.

When someone was newly diagnosed with HIV, I'd tell them the scientific truth: that in any epidemic there were a percentage who survived. Any one patient might be on the positive side of the statistical bell curve. There was always a chance, I would tell my patients, there was always a possibility they would be one of those to survive. At this point in my career, I'd only seen two long-term survivors, and one of them was me. Nonetheless, the hope I encouraged in my patients, I didn't entertain in myself. To give myself hope felt too much like I was fooling myself. Was I to be the exception, after all? Unlikely. If I had any number of malignancies, I calculated, my odds would have been better.

Would he have been one to actually survive the epidemic? Had I projected my own personal hopelessness onto Jerry and walked him to the edge where he didn't belong?

MARK RAUCH
"SURROUNDED BY LOVE"

In the last week of his life, my patient, Mark Rauch, wrote this letter to my team and me. From his hospital bed, and in his great illness, concentrating on and writing this must have been a colossal burden. But one morning on rounds that last week, he carefully handed this to me. I knew my parents understood that I practiced medicine, but I doubted they realized the scope of my work. I mailed them a copy of his letter followed by a note:

> The first time I was hospitalized I watched a lot of television. Most of it was dreadful. One show I enjoyed was "All in the Family." To be most precise, I enjoyed watching Edith. In hospitals there is much time to think and I thought about why I was so affected by this character called Edith. She wasn't pretty, or smart, or witty. She accomplished nothing that history would record. Her days were spent caring for her family.
>
> Edith cared. Edith did more than care, Edith loved. That was what made her real for me. She had that which can create paradise out of hell; she had that without which all is awful—she loved uncritically all who came into her life.
>
> Edith was only a character on a show, but I've known people like her. And it is to these people I wish to say "Thank you." You have comforted me in my despair, washed me, combed my hair, done my laundry. The world may never know of your kindness, but I know, and when I stand before God, your names will echo through the throne room

in praise until all the angels take up the cry, then will the universe tremble, and in its secret places write your names, but nowhere will they be engraved more deeply than in my heart.

You had but little you could give, yet you gave it. Great achievements were beyond you, yet you waged endless war against despair and fear. The get well card, the phone call, the visit you made, changed my life. I do not exaggerate. I could be dying alone, hopeless and unloved. Because of you, I die surrounded by love and I die loving you—the unseen saints of this earth.

You have comforted me, now may I comfort you. Pain shall pass, grief shall be forgotten. Love endures, and one day, be assured, the circle will be unbroken. Lift up your hearts.

Mark E. Rauch
Summer 1954—Autumn 1988

Dear Mom & Dad,
Mark died under my care Nov. 16 and wrote this letter to his doctors before he passed away (the dates at the bottom are his own). This is what I do. This is what I do for a living. I love you both. —Andrew

On the day that Mark died, I happened to have been kept at the hospital longer than usual. I was awaiting the arrival of a patient who needed to be admitted but who was delayed, and another patient who required a check-up following a particularly thorny procedure. Mark had pulmonary KS and, once chemotherapy and steroids had proven ineffective, he had decided that there should be no efforts to revive him once he passed. He was extraordinarily well-liked on the Immunosuppression Unit and he knew that such efforts would have been pointless, as well as tremendously upsetting for the nursing staff. He had made himself a DNR—a "do not resuscitate." That's the kind of person Mark was.

I happened to have been at the nursing station when his nurse came to me and told me that she expected him to leave us soon; within minutes, she thought. His lover had been called, but he was across town and wouldn't be there for at least half an hour. My second charge, I decided, would wait and I walked into Mark's room. It was odd to be able to approach him without ventilator paraphernalia and tubes obstructing his face and with the room now quiet, rid of the beeps and buzzes of the ventilator and his cardiac monitor. His ribs were visible and on his thin, thin chest, among the many angry, purple KS lesions, were the reddened circles where the cardiac monitoring pads had been. I had placed him on a morphine drip, both to ease his pain and to lessen any terror of "air hunger" he might experience. His breathing had become, ominously, subdued as he no longer battled to coax air into lungs too stiff and scarred to function. When he heard footsteps in the room, he opened his eyes. As I walked over and sat down in a chair next to his bed, his gaze followed me. I greeted him and made some irreverent remark about his needing to get out more. He smiled; he was amused. He closed his eyes. We sat there, the two of us, for no more than three minutes. He opened his eyes and turned his gaze towards me. He was too weak to turn his head. He was no longer capable of speech, in fact his lips barely moved as he mouthed the words: "thank you." He closed his eyes, and Mark Rauch left the room.

My mother had been a school teacher and principal and therefore, at one point, she had been the feared creature lurking in the principal's office; my father had been an engineer who worked on missiles for the US government, a genuine rocket scientist. But no one in our immediate or extended family had been a physician. They were as proud of my being a doctor as I was of my school-principal mother and my "rocket scientist" dad. My parents knew, of course, that I was HIV-positive and that I exclusively treated AIDS patients, though discussing the specifics of my work with them would have been unkind and unwanted.

My dad was not a man who kept things; he was not a "pack rat." In many ways, when it came to individual items, I found him frustratingly unsentimental. When my mother passed in 2009, I became irritated with him concerning those things of my mother's that he had discarded which I would have dearly loved. So it was with more than a little surprise that, as I sorted through his things after his death, I came upon this letter from Mark and my postscript.

Apparently Mark's letter had been as meaningful for him as it was for me.

PHYSICIANS, NOT PRIESTS

Most of my patients knew their fate as soon as they received an AIDS diagnosis (the formal diagnosis of AIDS, at the time, required both a positive HIV antibody test as well as an opportunistic infection or T-cells below 200), but a number of them had lived in isolation from others with the disease and were unacquainted with the illness. I knew that it was best to inform these men of their diagnoses as soon as possible since their learning this from some overheard, casual comment would have been brutal. To keep the patient uninformed, or half-informed, was tantamount to a lie that would have made it impossible to create a real connection. Besides, withholding or delaying information would have been an arrogant act of condescension as it assumed they were unable to process the information.

When it came to supplying the necessary details about their prognoses, I saw my function as sometimes, as nearly, that of a technician plainly giving unadulterated test results. (Precise life-span was obviously unknown and therefore avoided as much as possible.) In the beginning of my practice, I worried that I destroyed hope when I delivered the necessary information. But I found that whatever hope may have been lost and no matter the initial devastation, men who had more facts faced their end better in the long run—they seemed to experience less crippling terror and depression than I might have expected. I saw that embracing clear truth gave them an opportunity to face the totality of their lives and reach past a point of old grudges and allow forgiveness. Informing my patients was better than not; knowing was better than not knowing.

And if a patient remarked on his personal beliefs, if he introduced the subject, I would encourage him to elaborate on his spiritual views. My listening to the details of their convictions went a long way in making my patients feel understood and respected; moreover, actively listening expanded my grasp of their social web, their sensibilities, and their priorities. Conversation built connection. In being heard, my patients became more fully participants in medical and social decisions than just a knowledge of medical facts and statistics would have conveyed.

But there was another benefit, a personal benefit, in listening to my patients' thoughts and beliefs. I gained so much in vision and insights listening to these men who were closer to the edge than I was. With age one of the great lessons of my life is that we learn more from listening than talking. The actor Alan Alda once remarked that "Listening is being able to be changed by the other person." I learned that I could become so much more than who I was by listening.

In order to be free to discuss these issues without prejudice, however, I had to bury my own convictions and reject any temptation to introduce my own spiritual notions. If a patient feels that his doctor is uncomfortable discussing spiritual beliefs, dialogue will be damaged and support shortchanged. If I interrupted conversation, I may have made myself feel more comfortable, but not my patient.

I can't explain why some patients seemed to experience a greater measure of quiet, of calm, compared to those who dealt with more anguish and chaos. Other than working for connectedness, I certainly don't credit myself for any serenity my men may have achieved. I was merely a stepping stone on their journey. After all I was a physician, not a priest.

MORNING DEATH LISTS

After I had been at LMG for some time, we started making a list of those who had passed during the previous 24 hours. We were losing some two to three patients a week, sometimes two to three a day. To learn of someone's death by chance in an overheard conversation in the hall or a receptionist's remark on the telephone was excruciating in its surprise—the sudden news unnerving, startling us and distracting us from our work.

These deaths, while many if not most were expected, nevertheless wrought havoc with our emotions and concentration until it occurred to me to prepare a list to be available first thing in the morning. With this change in office procedure, each of us could read the list before work and, in our own way, mark the passing of those patients we had cared for. Even if I didn't recognize the name, it was likely I had seen the person in the office or hospital. On occasion, when I knew a week was particularly heavy in losses, I would come into the office a half hour or so early. There would be bustling activity in the front reception area, but not in the back doctors' lounge (a 15' by 15' corner office with a large table in the center nearly filling the room). Sometimes another doctor had arrived before, but usually I would come in sufficiently early to find the lounge deserted and quiet. I would search out that solitary page before the sounds of the office grew to a distraction—perhaps I would ask one of the receptionists to print it if it wasn't already.

Once I had the list, in the conference room I would brace myself and then take a quick glance at the number of names. Afterwards I would read each entry more carefully. Perhaps it was a patient of mine, perhaps it was someone I had consulted on days before, perhaps I had only seen them in the waiting room... but I knew them. The names better known would feel like a blow to my face. It was a rare day, however, that I would tear up—there were patients to be seen, other physicians to consult and lab reports to evaluate. But when the week's losses were especially numerous, or my connection to particular patients more intimate, I would leave the lounge and retreat into an empty exam room where I wouldn't be seen or disturbed and silently stare at the single white page heavy with names and, now, memories.

HARRY JOHNSON
A PATIENT'S FUNERAL

During those years I attended only one funeral of a patient. I had known Harry Johnson better than most and I felt compelled to say goodbye. The world had lost someone valuable when it lost Harry and I wanted the opportunity to mark the sad passing with those who loved him. Harry and his partner, David, had many friends and his parents and sister had been wonderfully supportive—it was to be a large funeral. Once I arrived at the church, I was startled to find myself in a sea of black dresses and dark suits. I didn't own a suit and I cursed my lack of planning; I was an AIDS doctor after all, it was absurd for me not to own a black funeral suit.

I sat on the aisle in the back row. There were a number of other patients there, but my presence was noticed only by one or two. I was struck by a paranoid, fleeting thought that somehow I would be identified as responsible for Harry's death.

In the center of a busy hallway in the North Hollywood Hospital, a patient's brother had once screamed that I'd killed his brother (by ordering a C.T. scan). This same brother had been homophobic toward the patient and routinely excluded him from family gatherings. It was my sad experience that frequently those who were the most critical of a patient's care were actually the most distanced. It is often the uninvolved mother, the critical brother, the judgmental father, the hyper-religious sister who criticizes a patient's care the most. I don't want to undervalue this man's grief, but this kind of reaction—usually on a lesser scale—was not uncommon in some family members.

But I knew, of course, Harry's family had loved him profoundly and I had treated him until there had been nothing more to do. As those present, perhaps 200, took their seats, I realized I was feeling uncomfortable and it had nothing to do with my clothing. I was troubled by the knowledge that I knew Harry far more intimately than many of those sitting in the pews. I had been with him through his presenting pneumonia and had identified the first lesion on his back as KS. I was there when he was tormented by thoughts of the grief he would cause those who loved him. I had been there when David pulled me out into a hospital hall and wept with his impotence and fatigue. I had known Harry very, very well in the last few months of his life—I was part of this group of mourners but strangely not. In spite of the deepest emotional connection, or because of it, I was outside this group of grieving people.

Somewhere in the service the reverend asked for anyone who had something to say, a memory perhaps, to stand and speak. Without a significant pause, several people got up and shared a memory aloud and I was surprised to learn of several details of his life I hadn't known. Finally there was a pause as the reverend waited for others to speak. The seconds seemed like minutes as I wrestled with myself whether I should stand and speak. There was so much that could be said: from Harry's courage to his love for David. But this was not about me, I reasoned—the attention was to be on Harry's life. I imagined my mother, however, who delighted in recounting drama and who would have reported how touching it was for the doctor himself to stand and speak. These feelings finally won out and just as I was about to stand, the interval ended. Part of me was relieved as I am not a public speaker, but another part was disappointed that my hesitation would mean Harry's gathered friends and relatives would not hear my few remarks, my few observations. And his mother wouldn't be able to say afterwards that even his doctor had stood to eulogize her son.

CANCER AT THE FRONT DOOR

In September of 1990, Jack developed a painless lesion in the back of his throat which he felt when he swallowed. I wish I had accompanied him to UCLA hospital the day he was examined, but the fact was that the problem didn't register with me, somehow, that it could have been something serious. It should have—we had known since his pneumonia in 1987 that he was immunocompromised and therefore my tranquility was rooted in denial. For me it was unthinkable that Jack might be up against one of those punishing diseases I saw in my office every day.

When he returned I was in my upstairs study—my "man-cave"—when I heard him slam the door. "I have cancer," I heard him yell. There was neither a remark before nor after. Just "I have cancer." I ran down the stairs. Yes, I had heard correctly. I could see the shock on his face as I had heard it in his voice. There was no manufactured distress that day, no faux horror to break the deathly seriousness of the moment as there had been at S.F. General those years before. This felt more serious than that, as it was. He didn't bawl then, his face didn't crinkle into a mask of play weeping as it did when he was clowning. Rather, his face remained motionless as tears silently wet his cheeks.

Jack "clucked," in his normal fashion meaning "this is what it is and I'll have to get used to it."

"Hey," I said. "This isn't all there is, there are things we can do." I grabbed his neck, and pressed my forehead to his.

After nine months of chemotherapy, Jack passed away no more than 10 feet from where we stood that day.

TOM JENNINGS
"IT'S NOT SUPPOSED TO HAPPEN
TO A DOCTOR"

I was interviewed in the fall of 1990, anonymously, for an article that appeared in the October 7, 1991, *L.A.C.M.A. Physician* (Los Angeles County Medical Association periodical). Tom Jennings was the author of the article entitled "It's Not Supposed to Happen to a Doctor." In it, I said I expected to be out of my practice in two years, dead in four. I told him, "What I've come to realize is that this is a lethal disease and it's going to take my life." But I also expressed surprise that I was doing so well. The CDC study, in which I remain an active subject, sees me about three times a year. (At least when they have federal funding.) A few years later, one of the researchers who was examining me suggested that my strain of HIV could be particularly weak; this may or may not be so, but what I did have was a missing CCR5 gene—an absence found most often in those of Northern European descent. In most people, this gene produces proteins on the surface of lymphocytes which effectively work as one of several "doors" for HIV entry. Without that gene's proteins, my lymphocytes have one less point of entry for the virus. There are still many other points of entry for the virus, obviously, so I am not immune.

Tom Jennings began his interview:

"Physicians seemed to have it all. He was young, he had a lucrative practice—and he had HIV. Now he talks, anonymously, about fear and prejudice in the medical community, and how that attitude must change."

Here are a few of the comments I made:

"I have seen many nurses and even physicians treating their HIV-positive patients in an inappropriate manner. I've seen nurses gown up and put on gloves to simply interview an AIDS patient. That is very distressing to the patient and is not based on scientific fact, but strictly on emotions. That does nothing for the patient's sense of well being and self respect...

"It makes me furious when I hear people like Senator Jesse Helms saying that spending for AIDS is out of proportion to other life-threatening illnesses. What he fails to take into account, even if he ignored the human cost and only looked at economics, is the man-years that are lost when a young person dies rather than an elderly person. If a grandmother who has heart failure dies, although it's tragic in its own right, society is not losing the productivity a 35-year old has to offer...

"I believe that HIV will eventually be curable and even prevented with vaccines. When that will happen, I don't know. I'm pessimistic that I will live to see it happen. Like I tell my patients: hope for the best, plan for the worst."

OUR DENIAL

Although we talked about our visits to the chemotherapy clinic and my anti-nausea formula, in that last year I took my cues from Jack and didn't discuss his death. Nor did we talk about any doubts he may have had about the chemotherapy he took for the last nine months of his life. He never asked me the percentage of those treated who survived long-term. (In those years, almost all patients with HIV-related non-Hodgkins lymphoma succumbed well within the first year.) When he was first hospitalized with PCP in San Francisco, he listened quietly when his father pressed him to do physical exercises, but he knew that his was a far more serious disease than could be treated by simple bed exercises. Despite Jack's opting for every medical treatment available, his clucking revealed his growing pessimism.

I spent much of my professional energies helping others work through their denial. It seemed that once the energy supporting denial was refocused, my patients frequently had more honesty and forgiveness with their loved ones and often a less troubled end. Randy Shilts, the great chronicler of the epidemic, wrote that his life was finished without being complete—my goal was to assist as many as I could in making their lives complete. It was the paradox of my life that as my practice became increasingly specialized in helping patients accept reality and walking with them the last steps of their lives, I didn't find this kind of success at home. But the truth was that I didn't employ all of my abilities; I simply couldn't be Jack's physician. People frequently lose their professional strengths once they're no longer functioning in their usual capacity and this was what occurred with me. For I was not his physician—I was his husband—and I simply didn't fit or want another role. The reality was I had my own denial and he may well have received signals from me that denied his mortality; I had, after all, conjured a thousand ways for him to survive. Engulfed by his own denial, I wanted to believe that in his preternatural innocence, in his tenacious happiness, he would survive. So in addition to my professional limitations, I wrestled with my own personal reluctance to accept the inevitable.

The day before he died he asked me what drug we would use next. As a doctor I said nothing, as a husband I told the lie that there was yet another option. But there was no remaining treatment.

MAKING A HOSPITAL ROOM HOME

Each time Jack was hospitalized I bought a poster for him and had it professionally framed—a serene print, something full of colors that soothed the eye and heart. It would be a finished piece of art, attractive enough to hang in our home. But first it would keep him company in the hospital, something to look at that wasn't institutional. I would hang it in his room, nailed to the wall, regardless of the nurses' protestations or hospital regulations. One of these would find a home on a wall in each facility, under harsh lighting, among voices of appeal and acquiescence in the early morning hours and there in the late afternoon hours when the sunlight is harsh and unrelenting and then again before dusk fell. He would have something homey then and something of me to tell him he wasn't alone whether it be three in the morning or three in the afternoon.

I always feared, for some reason now lost or never understood, that Jack might pass in the afternoon hours. Although it'd be more difficult to be with him at two or three a.m., it is more expected somehow, more seemly, for death to occur in the night.

When he came home there would be something new to hang in the house. Perhaps it was like a child mollified with candy after the doctor's poking and prodding—morphed into something more adult, more permanent. After its time on the hospital wall, the artwork would stay with us and I'd make room for it somewhere at home. So Jack would be wheel-chaired out of the hospital with a carefully-framed print balanced on his knees—a small reward for the travails of his latest hospitalization.

BOOKS, BARS AND BLUES

Jack had chemotherapy every Thursday until the last few weeks of his life when all treatment was futile. In my overheated schedule as physician and primary caregiver, this was one of the two days in my week that belonged to me. At LMG I changed my schedule to Monday through Wednesday and Friday and Saturday. In addition I served as on-call physician one week out of every four. On the weekends the on-call designate covered all hospitalized patients with their greater medical complexity and considerable demand for consultation with specialists, as well as meetings with families and significant others. During the last year of my practice, I found myself being asked to do more and more hospital work as opposed to clinic work. I was keenly aware of how little we knew about the disease and it was this insecurity that fueled my professional drive and attention to detail. We had a reputation for treating AIDS patients well—not just from a cutting edge, up-to-the-minute scientific perspective, but also from a psychological/emotional point of view. "You don't have to *be* the smartest doctor, you just have to *hire* the smartest doctor," Fred would repeat. But Fred and Vincent had another reason for increasingly shunting me to the hospital. My colleagues could depend on my ability to treat people medically—and emotionally—at the very worst moments of their lives. In our efforts to connect with people, our most powerful tool is empathy and my life story and my own HIV status, while undisclosed, gave me an empathy which translated into an ease in achieving this all-important connectedness. My history and HIV status wasn't known or stated explicitly, but my patients nevertheless knew we stood shoulder to shoulder: "You are not alone," "We're in this together." So I was spending more and more of my time on hospital rounds and taking weekend calls—juggling technical detail and despondency.

I was incredibly grateful that there was not a word of complaint from anyone in the office when I began to take every Thursday off to be with Jack for his chemotherapy. We would get up together on those days and have a breakfast of something bland like yogurt and cereal. I would have my coffee and he would have his tea just the way he liked it. I'd carefully watch the clock so we wouldn't be rushing as we drove to UCLA hospital. There we would park in their below-ground parking and find our way to the outpatient treatment. After signing in and sitting down in an attractive waiting room, we would search the tables for anything which would distract us a bit from the other patients waiting for chemotherapy and our approaching treatment. During those first months the sight of our thin co-travelers with their haunted eyes and tell-tale turbans and baseball caps would hit us like a bucket of cold water. But after some five or six weeks of therapy, the shock of their appearance melted away and we began seeing them as the three-dimensional people they were.

Jack, who found silence to be deadly and individual relationships engrossing, would frequently strike up a conversation and find hope in the worst case scenarios. I, on the other hand, found it difficult to relax and challenging to engage other patients in conversation. No matter. Although occasionally nervous, Jack fulfilled his role as the consummate party thrower. The eternal mingler, he would tease out their stories while, unexpectedly, keeping silent about much of his own. A beautiful 23-year-old woman with brain cancer answered Jack's sympathetic questioning, "Oh, I was cancer-free for six months and I'm back again." She produced pictures of her cat playing, and reported that the cat was pregnant and she hoped to live long enough to see the birthing. The others in the waiting room were a different group of people: middle-aged women with breast cancer, less well-kept older men with prostate cancer, and the occasional young person in their early 20s or 30s with a heavy metal band displayed on their T-shirt. This last group, the younger ones, would haunt my thoughts for days after we were back at home—they had probably seen the best days of their lives.

I was a little surprised to see that most patients came alone, but there were many who came accompanied. Some barely spoke, but they each had their own life story, and through the random remarks and sometimes serious discussions we caught glimpses of how they viewed and managed their lives. It was a time together that could make us feel good about ourselves, our doctors and our conditions one week, and then desperately depressed the next. I would like to say that because of my daily work, I wasn't negatively affected by this group with different cancers and different attitudes, but their haggard, run-down appearance did everything but convince me that cures were right around the corner for any of us. And once it became clearer that Jack wasn't doing as well as we hoped, he slipped into the role of happy interviewer less and less.

When they called Jack's name, we'd walk into the chemotherapy suite and I would sit him down in one of the hyper-comfortable lounge chairs which UCLA had specifically for this purpose. Each high-backed chair was its own little alcove, its own niche, although there was little actual privacy owing to the constellation of some 20 other chairs on each side and across the large room; but it was a cheerful place with big picture windows looking out onto a green lawn. One could not ask for better nurses—they were patient, competent and reasonably cheerful. I would hold Jack's hand while they found a cooperative vein and sit there while the medication dripped into him. Always the comedian, Jack would make comic observations of the nurses attending him, sometimes within their hearing, sometimes not. But the real targets of his remarks, albeit unknown to them, were the other patients in their own separate lounge chair-cubicles surrounding ours. Those around us were seldom party to his insightful remarks or his uncanny witticisms, but had his observations been overheard, I suspect most patients as well as bystanders would have laughed in recognition and agreement. Though they may not have known it, Jack was an ally.

I deeply appreciated UCLA's gesture of providing something of the natural world to enjoy. Those facing severe illnesses can enjoy so much from an open window or an open door. It seems the valuable effects of nature are multiplied in those debilitated sick who face the sterile world of windows that don't open and rain that can't be heard. Sometimes when we think we have nothing to offer the dying, it can be such an easy thing to simply take someone outside. Getting outdoors into nature, even if it is just the grass of a backyard, can help calm our fears and refocus our energies. One of my patient's friends once took him on a short trip to a small nearby park and, even on this man's deathbed, he mentioned the beauty of this park and spoke repeatedly about his buddy's thoughtfulness and efforts.

Music, too, is of tremendous value—many people have noticed that it uncovers and articulates those emotions which need to be expressed and it may be one of the few pleasures that one is still able to remember and experience. Music can give us access to words and worlds that we may forget in the all-consuming centripetal focus of fatal illness. In my own life auditory memories from long ago can comfort me in ways both mysterious and intense. Oliver Sacks writes of "a deep and mysterious paradox here, for while music makes one experience pain and grief more intensely, it brings solace and consolation at the same time." A symphony conductor of ours battled near constant hysteria without music—but once we arranged for a boombox in his room, his anxiety drifted away. Many of our patients responded to music with a serenity they seemed to find in nothing else. This was more frequently the case in Los Angeles —perhaps because my patients seemed to be more engaged with music and those technical maneuvers needed to get it in their rooms.

Most people fear pain and loss of autonomy when they face fatal illness. While I could lessen the universal fear of pain at the end of a person's life, loss of independence was something I couldn't necessarily address because everyone's situation was so different. Sometimes it meant ensuring they were receiving as much help as possible from the medical system and insurance company. Occasionally it was helpful to frame extra work as a gift that the loved one was gladly giving, or that the added assistance was more effort than it appeared (rarely the case). There were times when receiving help from someone could be understood as metaphysical lessons in humility, or in providing such opportunity for spiritual growth for those who are helping—the last being more difficult for everyone to accept.

Although it may seem obvious, one of the most important things I learned in serving my brothers was that our goal must always be to help people live their lives as fully, as unencumbered, by their disease as long as is possible.

I will never know for sure if Jack was one of those extraordinarily few patients who seem to simply not get nauseous from the potent drugs he was receiving, but he never once threw-up during the months of his intravenous chemotherapy. About an hour before he was to receive the IV infusion, I would give him some medications from a recipe all my own. Unfortunately I can no longer remember it entirely but it had acetaminophen, a couple of different drugs in the Valium family, as well as compazine (at that time a first-line nausea suppressant) and a bit of anti-histamine. It is true he could remember little of those Thursdays for medications in the diazepam family are well-known to produce anterograde amnesia. But the fact that Jack never experienced even one sustained bout of nausea remains one of my most gratifying successes. Afterwards, as we drove home, Jack would doze in the car. Towards the end of his life he'd need help walking from the garage to our condo, but once there the exhausting chemotherapy would combine with my recipe and he would crawl into bed and fall fast asleep, his face relaxed, his body finally at rest.

As he became more ill and slept through Thursday nights, those hours after chemotherapy became my own, my one night when I could go out as Jack slept soundly. I once overheard Fred Lawrence talking to a straight friend about a gay couple, Bradly and Tom, the latter being in intensive care for prolonged periods. During the day, Bradly would be with Tom constantly. But at night, while his partner slept, Bradly would make his own rounds, going to bars and baths. The friend, hearing this, complained about Bradly's "infidelities." Fred's response was quick and unequivocal: he pointed out Bradly's devotion to Tom, his constant presence at the bedside while his partner was awake, his tenacious loyalty throughout the long and draining illness. Who was to judge this person or his ethics? Such perspective could have applied to me—my Thursday nights could also have been condemned—for as Jack slept deeply those nights, I would take a few hours for myself. I spent my time in bars, drinking little, as was my usual, but socializing and diving into AIDS fund-raisers. For caregivers, time away is vital—for an army cannot fight without clothing, food, and rest.

Besides my Thursday night escapes, I found books to be reassuring. Reading medical journals was a necessity which left me without the spare time or focus to read novels or other books of length. But economy of words made poetry and plays accessible: I read, among others, John Donne, W. H. Auden, Thom Gunn, the plays of Tennessee Williams and Henrik Ibsen and "coffee table" books of the architecture of Frank Lloyd Wright and the Austrian

Wiener Werkstätte design movement. When we traveled to Europe in 1989, I lugged along a far-too-heavy volume of my favorite poet, Edna St. Vincent Millay. I do not fit so readily into the e-society of today as I find a book's physicality is part of its appeal; the sturdiness of books promises survival in the face of inconstant electronics. Something in life, my books told me, could evade obliteration. But books and bars weren't my only escape. Every Sunday night there was a Rhythm & Blues TV program which drew my attention and anticipation. Music gave me solace in demonstrating the stability of ongoing life and that permanence of auditory pleasure. Occasionally the past joy of an old song or musical phrase could mysteriously transform the emotions I was experiencing into a pleasure akin to that which I had felt long before. Books, bars and blues. These were a few comforts in a brutal routine.

THE TRIP-WIRE FOR TEARS

Jack was never much of a tea drinker, but over the course of his treatment, his tastes changed and he began drinking tea. UCLA hospital couldn't necessarily give its patients longer lives, but it could provide them an extravagant selection of teas. Towards the end of his life now, he looked pale, gaunt and frail; he was weak and irritable, and his impatience frazzled our bond. But every time I saw him in those days, my heart was scratched with the realization that he would soon be gone. How would I live without him? I am an introvert by nature, an extrovert by necessity; being around people drains me of energy, being alone charges my batteries. That is not to say that I, and other introverts, cannot rise to the occasion and be great successes at a party. But life is easier for an introvert when they can push an extrovert partner forward to "do the heavy lifting."

On a particularly frustrating day, Jack didn't like his tea, which he blamed on me as I was serving as tea barista. We walked into the suite, more slowly than we ever had before, and once Jack was seated I traveled to its other end where the refreshments were. I had prepared his tea according to his specific instructions which were, I thought, maddeningly idiosyncratic and needlessly stringent. Perhaps he was exercising the only control he had, but my concoction was refused four times that day. Seeing Jack in that condition, however, defused any impatience or frustration I might have had. I was much aware that there, but for the grace of god, go I. This was not as hypothetical as it may seem: I was constantly aware that the virus was eating away at my immune system and could turn in a heartbeat and leave me with the same malignancy. It is easier to walk in someone else's shoes when your own instep is being measured.

As I was walking back and forth to the "Refreshment and Welcoming" counter, another nurse, who wasn't Jack's, noticed my meticulous preparation of his tea. She came to me, as I was pouring the hot water, and told me that Jack could not have had a better partner. It is an odd phenomenon—under great emotional stress we can plow along with whatever task we're given and we carefully hold our emotions in check until, often by accident, the beauty of our actions are recognized and an unseen psychological trip-wire is snagged. For me that day all the frustration and grief were released and I broke down sobbing. I don't recall the particular nurse's name, I may have never known it, but she knew mine.

GEORGE KRIVACEK AND LLOYD BURR
DOUBLE TRAGEDY

Lloyd Burr eventually got a police "ankle monitor" as a result of a DUI or some liquor store altercation—it was never clear which. In any case, he was confined to the house as a measure of public safety and George had to be the one to buy Lloyd liquor as he was the only one able to leave their house. At several points through the years, George had threatened to break off their relationship if Lloyd wouldn't stop drinking. Finally George had refused to buy any more alcohol—leaving Lloyd at home to navigate as best he could. Under the strain of being HIV-positive and cut off from liquor, Lloyd had taken a shotgun and fired it at his head. He'd done it in the living room of their home—only a few feet from where those dinners with the four of us had taken place. The county coroner had just left the house with Lloyd's body, George spoke in shock. Would I come over and help him clean up?

Looking back now it seems horribly absurd for the two of us to be cleaning up the blood, hair and bits of body tissue which remained. I simply didn't know one could hire professionals who are trained for such things as this. Upon arriving at the house and finding the inconceivably horrendous remains of human despair, I know I offered to clean up everything alone, without George's ashen-faced help. I should have insisted that he leave while I dealt with the scene of horror. But it was a time when many of us found ourselves doing things we never imagined.

But as I look back, there was a sacredness to our cleaning: a piety, a devotion, perhaps a penance, in our quiet work that day and well into the night. There was also a farewell, far more prolonged than funerals provide, for those of us remaining on this planet. We are so different, one from another, in spite of our similar anatomy and circuitry, that I am sometimes amazed that we can understand each other at all. That it is even possible that we can speak the same language. And in this unknowable difference in finite and fragile muscle, bone and blood, who are we to judge our brothers? In that day, in that time, we took care of each other, buried each other and mourned each other. In the onslaught of so many deaths, the societal conventions normally guiding us were irrelevant. Each of us could be struck down at any minute, as if by gunfire, as if in war, while society functioned normally around us. The San Francisco gay newspaper, *Bay Area Reporter*, filled two pages every Thursday with obituaries and we read in wonder and dread who had died the preceding week. The paper, early on, was forced to make strict rules for obituary submission in order to have enough space for them all. Meanwhile in the mainstream culture, news of our devastation remained minimized or absent. In such a world of imminent death and relentless loss, in this subculture of grief, we made our own rules and rituals of death as best we could. It was in this spirit of not fully knowing the human kneeling beside me that I didn't push George to let me do the whole clean-up job by myself.

* * *

It was during the last month of my practice that George Krivacek came to me with a vial of "Chinese Compound Q." The top of the vial wasn't capped in a sterile manner and I asked him what he wanted me to do with the amber liquid.

"Inject it into me."

"George, to start with, it's not a sterile solution in a sterile vial. Secondly, we don't know what it is and we have no idea what it will do."

Although AZT had sickened him beyond tolerance and he'd stopped it, his health didn't seem to be declining. He was thin, but not emaciated. Now I echoed my intensive care attendings: who knew when a cure would be discovered? It could be tomorrow, I said. He waved away such a possibility.

"It's doing amazing things according to underground

druggies. Some say it's a cure that the US government just doesn't want us to have," he replied.

Every once in a while, I'd encounter someone who saw the world through the clouded gauze of conspiracies: in a world turned upside down with confusion and helplessness, forbidden knowledge gives us feelings of certainty, control and comfort, and since these individuals believed authorities couldn't be trusted, people had to find the truth on their own. Now he had fallen into the conspiracy theory that the only truly effective treatment came from possessing secret knowledge that "they" didn't want us to have—a conviction that access to concealed information makes us, somehow, safer.

"Ah, George, we've been over this. There's no one in the U.S. government smart enough to come up with HIV. And there's nothing, really, they don't want you to have; if anything, they don't care about you."

"Andrew, you know I love you, but you can be very naïve about the government and what it's doing." He threatened to inject it himself at home, alone, in non-sterile conditions. He believed Compound Q was a wonder drug, but he preferred to have me there. He trusted me, he said. George was unshakeable.

It was with a heavy heart that I took the vial and irradiated it at our hospital. I knew there was no way I could inject him there; I had the hospital's legal standing to protect as well as my license. Looking back, at the least I should have had a chemical analysis performed. If I refused him, would he really inject himself? We drove to his house in the Valley, just the two of us in my car. I entreated him again not to go through with it. I echoed my Intensive Care attendings: who knew when a cure would be discovered? It could be tomorrow, I said. He waved away such a possibility.

"If we're going to do it, and we are, let's do it," he said.

He lay down on the living room couch, with Lloyd's blood still staining the floor beneath us, steps away from the dining table where the four of us had eaten. He lay back. I filled the syringe from the vial and prepared his arm.

"One last chance, George, to say no. We don't know what this is."

"Just do it."

It was to be one of the great mistakes of my life.

I planted the needle and injected the yellowish fluid. Within a few minutes he blanched and threw up. I dialed 911.

George Krivacek was never the same. His unconsciousness in the first few hours grew into an agitated coma—a condition that can appear to an onlooker as if the individual is having horrible nightmares but cannot awaken. After nearly two weeks of intensive care, he finally awoke. Dreadfully gaunt when he was discharged a few weeks later, the sparkle had left his eyes.

Even if I were just being a responsible friend, I should have checked up on him, but at that time Jack was still living and my mind was completely taken up with the hurricanes of the day. I heard of his passing in some off-the-cuff remark by a mutual friend a few months later. And so it went.

Someone reading my account of those years may be misled by my frequent reference to bars. In fact I was never much of a drinker, but these establishments were much more than places of commerce. They were where the community congregated, they were where our families were. Bars were where we met new people and bumped into the old, where we had events like leather and drag shows, AIDS' auctions and contests and raffles. Some of us came from places where being out meant you had a target on your back. We had come from the Midwest and the Great Lakes and Texas and Indiana. We had come from places where it wasn't safe to be gay. Where being gay could get you thrown out of your house when you were 15, into fights with guys who had to prove something, or into high schools where you would overhear remarks by girls who giggled. Places like Wyoming, where you could get beaten up and tied to a wooden fence with barbed wire. The world slaps around black kids and Mexican kids and Asian kids when they're out of the house, but in a way I envied them: they had homes where they could go at night and be with people like them, houses of shelter, homes of refuge. Most of us, some by our own making, had residences where we were just as isolated inside as we were outside. Some of us never had places where you were home. Bars were places like that for us—the children of Hamelin. These were locations where clocks froze and the ill and painfully thin could walk among us without question or comment. Men I met, men I knew, men that were my patients—none ever asked me opinions concerning treatment or prognosis. Everyone understood that these were places of refuge from the inferno; we left our griefs and our illnesses at the door. Here we lived in the moment. Among our brothers.

In spite of this affable avoidance, I admit to having a daydream that, outside of the office or hospital, I would one day run into a patient whose care had been a satisfying success. With the majority of my patients dying, I developed a different vision. But in October of 1995 I ran into a former patient of mine, Richard Speakman. "That day in your office when you told me I was HIV-positive," he told me, "you had the broadest shoulders in the world."

His single sentence flooded that inner part of me which had grown arid with doubts concerning the value of the part I had played in the epidemic. Despite my best efforts, nearly all of my patients had passed away; what had all my efforts actually accomplished? I know that I had given many a bit of comfort and connection in their last days here with us, but it was nevertheless under my care that my patients had breathed their last. Our feelings are not easily-controlled bits of logic—the whipsaw of emotions occasionally catapulted my mind into the destructive dead-end of a binary world. The grace of running into a former patient was unlikely. Years later it was the internet that eventually led me to Richard's whereabouts: he had passed a year after our conversation.

Later, after Jack's death, I'd be out at a bar or store and meet some friend of a patient or a friend of someone I knew. Perhaps he was an intelligent or witty man—someone fun and lively, someone who could help lift me out of the morass of sadness and shut out the future I believed awaited me. Maybe we'd have a couple of beers together and share bits of our lives, but we'd carefully avoid any mention of AIDS, or sickness, or death. We'd exchange phone numbers or maybe not. But then in a couple months or so, I'd run into a mutual acquaintance of this new compatriot. "Hey, I met Mike, or Tom, or Jim the other day," I'd say and then hear the reply: "Oh, he died two weeks ago." By that time, we wouldn't say things like "Sorry to tell you" or "Didn't you know?" It was just a fact. One of many ordinary facts. One of many deaths.

DON WHITMAN
BACK AT WORK ON MONDAY

I saw Don Whitman for the first time in our offices on a Friday when he needed immediate hospitalization. He was slightly short of breath, coughing frequently, and on his lower chest exam I could hear constricted airways in both lungs. He was emaciated and displayed the hallmark seborrheic dermatitis between his eyes, on his forehead, in the creases around his nose. After this initial evaluation I admitted him to the hospital and started him on pentamidine even before his chest X-ray results were known.

When I next saw him he was on an oxygen mask and each of his arms had an IV line—one with pentamidine to fight his pneumonia and one for access and fluids. I asked him how he was doing and he replied that he was fine. While I puzzled over how to start the conversation, he spoke again. It was difficult to hear him over the hiss of the oxygen mask and the beeps of his finger oximeter. I leaned closer, now above him.

"What did you say, Don?"

"I need ..." he spoke through his breathlessness. "I need to be back at work on Monday."

The cognitive dissonance was striking. It was Friday and it was doubtful he would last a week. But his question informed me that, in spite of the objective clarity of his situation, he didn't understand what little time he had.

"Don," I started—but we were interrupted by the entrance of a nurse and a nurse's aid bringing him a meal he couldn't eat.

"Excuse me," I said, "we need a little time here." The irony of my words ricocheted in my head, behind my glasses. My eyes stayed on him as they left the room. "Don, you're very, very sick. You are dying. Do you have a partner or some close friends you can call to be with you?" I asked.

"Yes," he spoke between breaths, "I've got a buddy in West Hollywood and my sister is in Denver."

"You should call them right away because you need help."

Although his oxygen saturation fell through the night and into the next day, and I told him his life would soon be over, he didn't agree to "Do Not Resuscitate" orders. But he had called his friend and sister.

It was Dr. Mark Higgins, who eventually became my physician in San Francisco, who emphasized that it is essential to know the extent of a patient's interactions with people with AIDS—and therefore their grasp of the course of the disease itself. Evidently Don knew few, if any, people who had AIDS.

Don barely survived the weekend. He died Monday after a futile resuscitation attempt by the hospital doctors and nurses with the ubiquitous "crash cart." He had stepped off the earth only three days after his hospital admission.

FRED BECOMES ILL

About a year before I left the practice, Fred Lawrence hired two accomplished, published neurologists, one being Elaine Feraru, M.D. Shortly before disability forced me to leave LMG, the other neurologist resigned. Although his departure didn't affect me directly, it added a bit of uncertainty and instability to our office precisely when things were growing more difficult and unsteady for me. It was at this point Fred asked me to increase my hospital in-patient responsibilities, which meant dealing with more end-of-life issues than what was routinely found in our clinic.

It became apparent that I had a gift for assisting the dying. In helping those dying reach some relief in the last days or weeks of their lives, my work was appreciated not only by LMG, but also by physicians outside the group. Often unsure of optimum HIV care and uncomfortable with end-of-life issues, it wasn't unusual for doctors to transfer patients to the care of LMG. It is not exaggeration to say that Vincent and Fred hospitalized their patients under my care without concern—either for technical diligence or for emotional attention.

Several of my patients had meaningful, supportive relationships with their families and their lovers' families before their illnesses peaked. But it was my observation that if such a connection didn't already exist, such attachments rarely developed after one's illness showed itself. However, in a handful of situations where a bond had not previously been present, I witnessed patients and their families develop unexpected connections. These involved healing discussions in which disgust was ignored and old judgments abandoned. Often my brothers, in uncomfortable closets and ill-fitting disguises, had lived opaque lives viewed as impoverished and confusing by those with whom, in other galaxies, they might have had rich relationships. There was powerful beauty when an individual was at last seen as the three-dimensional person he had always been.

These events, although only a few, were bittersweet exercises in the establishment of connections between those who might have loved each other long before. I would like to be able to say that as time progressed I saw more and more relationships resolving in such circumstances, but from my observations they remained the exception. My impression has been that in the late 1990s such phenomena occurred with greater frequency, but I was not to witness such a revolution during my years of practice. The full weight of the epidemic had yet to swing society's judgments in our favor.

During the last months of my practice, I was assigned more hospital rounds and proportionally less office practice. Hospitalized patients are sicker, of course, and while I didn't mind expanding the technical side of care, their intense emotional demands began to take a toll on me. Lawrence Medical was truly accommodating in giving me every Thursday off in order to accompany Jack to chemotherapy at UCLA, and did so without complaint. But at that point caring for additional hospitalized patients was an emotional drain I could ill afford. I had given my ear and heart as best I could, but with some cost to myself. I had gone to three Goodbye Parties and one funeral and given my best care to dozens of others and I was learning that grief is cumulative: the death of even the least-known patient, transferred to me just hours before his demise, had weight. By postponing grief's full expression, I was only papering over what I would feel much more painfully later.

I began to forget the names of well-known patients. When on-call I had difficulty identifying the crux of patients' complaints. In order to jog my memory, I began to take home the charts of patients likely to call. I was losing sense of exactly when I had ordered what medication—especially those prescriptions I had phoned into the hospital or local pharmacies. The dosages of common medications began to slip my mind and I even began to lose that primitive, subconscious knowledge of which day of the week it is.

I was forgetting too much.

And then Fred Lawrence became ill. Due to the legal reasons I've described, we physicians did not inquire as to each other's HIV status. I didn't know the HIV status of other LMG doctors and they didn't know mine. Fred had begun practice in the relatively innocent days of mere STDs: gonorrhea, syphilis, chlamydia, non-specific urethritis, etc. When HIV emerged he rode the swell, as I did, of medical need. He was never board certified in a speciality, such as Family Practice, choosing instead to exit academia sooner rather than later and trust his own capabilities and entrepreneurial instincts. He had made the switch from easy, cookbook medicine to the obscure nuances and harsh realities of what was then one of the least understood diseases in medicine. And he had made the transition with flying colors. Now he himself was ill.

Our neurologist Elaine came to me in the Immunosuppression Unit of North Hollywood Hospital. I was taken aback when she took me into a small nursing supply room and closed the door. As she sought such privacy, I assumed yet another of the doctors or office staff had become ill or, in that brutal world of the 1980s and '90s, been found dead. It was the former, but the physician was Dr. Lawrence himself.

The space was small—it hadn't been designed to house people.

"Fred's sick," she said. "His chest X-ray is whited out." I was caught off-guard. Even though we were living in a world where death was a constant occurrence, my surprise was proportional to his emotional proximity.

"How long has he been sick?" I asked.

"He's had a non-productive cough for ten days, maybe two weeks," Elaine answered. "I need your help," she continued. "He refuses to come into the hospital. You know Fred, he insists on being treated at home."

I slowly digested the shock. He was a gay man active during the worst years of contagion and his illness should not have been a great surprise. But he was a doctor, and our training had taught us that, as physicians, we were indestructible. We didn't become sick. Our responsibilities and schedules had been such that anything approaching illness was simply rejected. Some of my colleagues obnoxiously embraced the "god complex" because what they considered superhuman had been expected—and attained. However, such convictions were as much myth as was Fred's health and immortality. His X-ray was snowing lethal white. He had *Pneumocystis* pneumonia.

The enemy was at the gate.

Fred's bed was a huge affair, with an enormous canopy from which Elaine had initially hung the bags of pentamidine before an IV pole arrived. As he felt comfortable with her, only once did I make the drive over to his house in the Hollywood Hills to hang a bag. But the shock of his illness was as profound as if I had diagnosed the infection in a lover; in the office, we were routinely losing members of our staff to illness, suicide, and mental issues due to the nature of our work. At home I was navigating the tortuous paths of Jack's medical schedules and his roller coaster of emotions while my hospital workload was increasingly weighted towards the most ill. Before Fred's diagnosis I had requested that I do less hospital work but with the loss of Dr. Olson and the other neurologist it was clear that working less, at that time, wasn't possible. I needed to round on more hospitalized patients.

MY LAST DAY IN PRACTICE

It had been a full week with a good number of patients in the hospital, many quite ill with three, in particular, who would certainly not survive longer than a few days. There had been a family conference scheduled for one of them. Work was increasingly demanding as my mind was clouded and I required extra effort to remember the details of those drugs we, in fact, used frequently. I was preoccupied with the death of our colleague Luke Olson, and the increase in work from his and Fred's absence had put Vincent, as well as the office staff, on edge.

While Jack's energy and mood rose and fell from day to day, his chemotherapy treatment had been a particular challenge. He hadn't experienced nausea or vomiting, but those mere possibilities paled in contrast to the actualities of those present. The body aches, headaches and overwhelming fatigue—the general discomfort—were beginning to weigh on him. Although I hadn't noticed evidence per se, I was beginning to feel that he and I were drifting apart as his illness began to take up more of his energies and attention. There was less enthusiasm as I walked in the door each night, fewer of his manufactured pratfalls; music and TV shows became more irritating than distracting as he sought the comfort of sleep.

It was a Saturday and the day was to be a full one. After rounding on hospitalized patients, I had a day of appointments waiting for me at the Wilshire office. Elaine was also seeing patients that day and she had asked me to go out to dinner with her that night.

Meanwhile I just wanted to lie down.

At the hospital, I reviewed my first patient's chart and then examined him. He was young, somewhere in his late 20s. Whatever his diagnoses were, John wasn't going to survive long and a discussion with his family was planned. We were soon gathered in one of the conference rooms and as we spoke of his imminent death, to my consternation I began to tear. I felt distant, emotionally detached, as if I were outside my body watching myself. My tears began to fall down my cheeks and obscure the chart. The family was grief-stricken over their son's approaching death but, it was easy to see, further confused and, I imagine, dismayed by their doctor's tears.

There are times when it is not necessarily bad for one's physician to cry. But this hadn't been one of those times; I had needed to be strong and confident and I hadn't been.

To worsen the situation, I hadn't remembered that there were two more family conferences scheduled in which similar outcomes were to be reviewed: the individual son or brother was unlikely to survive more than a few days. Each time I cried and each time it was inappropriate. I couldn't remember when I'd lost my composure this way. What was happening?

TO WORK OR TO LIVE

Although Elaine was wearing down my resistance, I continued to refuse dinner with her. I was bewildered over what had happened that morning—that and the fatigue of the day was at the heart of my refusal. I was feeling overwhelmed but simultaneously, without fully realizing it, oddly distanced. She must have seen the desperation just beneath the surface, for she wouldn't accept my refusal.

Over the course of dinner, I became the object of our mutual attention; I confessed my exhaustion and I reviewed the disturbing tears I had experienced at that morning's family meetings. Together we reviewed the trouble I was having remembering simple medications. I disclosed that I was HIV-positive—something I had never divulged to any physician with whom I was working. Elaine did not stay quiet: she interrupted several times to ask for pertinent details. How was I managing Jack and his malignancy? She was listening as a sympathetic friend, but she was also collecting data as a trained neurologist who specialized in HIV.

After considering the information she shocked me to my core, "You've got to quit."

What? She couldn't be serious! I contested her opinion. I said I was just exhausted, somewhat depressed and at most needed some time off. But in a few moments the hard realization hit me—*I had subconsciously been wishing I would contract pneumonia.* If I were ill, I could at last escape what had become a terrible, crushing burden. Tears of that morning became tears of that night.

"If you want to get sick, this is a disease that will give you what you wish for," she responded. "the practice will survive without you."

She was resolute. "Right now. Absolutely. You can't go back to work."

There were sirens in my head. I couldn't breathe.

Elaine was as wise as she was dispassionate. She was doing her job; it was a speech the both of us had given many times before. But this time I wasn't giving it, I was the one hearing it.

Usually a job is necessary to earn a living and, if one is fortunate, engage our minds and passions as it consumes our time. But for some a job is experienced as identity. For my physical and emotional health, to attain an untroubled, low-stress life, Elaine was voicing the unthinkable: I needed to leave this definition of myself behind. So it was during that dinner in a Studio City restaurant that it all came crashing down around my ears. For the second time in my life, I fought a battle to keep my profession. Although she thought there was a chance it was merely depression, she was doubtful. Just as before, this was a choice between preserving my career or preserving my life.

The sirens in my head suddenly went silent. The world stopped. I knew in that shattering instant that she was right. My survival trumped everything: freshman chemistry with the T.A. who spoke no English, the barely-managed terror of Organic Chemistry, the essays on political discourse, the hours of research, the mind-snapping tests, numberless discussions with professors, attendings, study groups; diligent patient examinations; the punishing enforced sleep deprivation of scores of on-call nights. Their hard-fought result was now to be relinquished.

Elaine had said it all: "If you want to be sick, this is a disease which will give you what you wish for." It was Saturday—I called Vincent and the wheels of my future began to realign.

As long as I had thought that my difficulties might be attributable to depression, I had something of a cushion from imagining my career was ended. While some HIV dementia was certainly possible, I held on to the hope my memory problems were due to simple depression. Neurologic testing in the days ahead would show that the source wasn't just depression, but principally complications of HIV encephalopathy—HIV impacting the functions of the brain. My career was over.

RESIGNING FROM
LAWRENCE MEDICAL GROUP

So it was in February of 1991 that my departure from medicine came. Jack was into month five of his chemotherapy at UCLA. We were losing about one patient every other day and I was caring for more and more hospitalized patients. Some end-stage patients from other practices were being transferred to LMG care and I was seeing them. Luke Olson, M.D., had been hospitalized and passed away the November before. Fred had just recovered from his own bout with PCP. And then there were the deaths of other Lawrence Medical staff; we had lost Mark, our office assistant, the preceding fall and another assistant, after a positive HIV test, had been found dead in his bathtub with his wrists slit; there was no suicide note. Our colleagues were fast becoming our patients. My discussion with Elaine had occurred two days before. It was time.

To All My Patients,
Effective February 4, 1991, I am taking an indefinite leave of absence from my responsibilities here at Lawrence Medical Group. In order to meet some challenges at home, and remain available for the future needs of our community, I am withdrawing from the practice for the time being. This has not been a particularly easy decision, but as I am sure one can readily understand, we are involved in a special work which occasionally requires special considerations. A great comfort to me is the knowledge that the care you receive here at Lawrence Medical is unsurpassed, unsurpassed not only in the sense of up-to-the-minute

technical sophistication, but also unsurpassed in the sense of providing this care in the context of human dignity and with the understanding of the paramount importance of the quality of life.

This context of care is an understanding of priorities which is identical to that which has always been my personal and professional goal.

I remain available to help smooth whatever difficulties this transition may represent for you and thank you, in advance, for your understanding and support. I will miss you all.

Sincerely Yours,
Andrew M. Faulk, M.D.

DEPARTURE FROM PRACTICE

My departure from medicine and the career I loved is a difficult story to tell. As an undergraduate at Columbia, I double-majored in pre-medicine and political science. I couldn't know what a career in medicine would mean but I did know the long march through medical school, internship and residency required years. I was a pauper while my graduated friends had jobs and incomes and girlfriends/boyfriends/spouses and children. Without these I felt like an adolescent, my social life had been frozen. I had had no time and no money and, quite narcissistically, I felt it.

After graduation from college, for a time I worked as a paralegal at the Wall Street law firm of White & Case. It was an important opportunity, for I witnessed an unnerving distillation of this profession. Those attorneys below the level of partner were demoralized and, to a person, passionately discouraged anyone from making law a career. I had never before, nor have I since, had a chair thrown at me, even by a patient lost in the throes of a psychiatric hurricane. Had there been any doubt before, there was none now. Attorneys were fighters; physicians were nurturers. My identity as the latter was now certain—I was a nurturer. In medicine I was needed, in law I would be superfluous. And a potential target for errant office furniture.

With my identity intimately tied to my work, it has been a strain to separate the two. In fact, should you ask those who love me, they would tell you it is an issue with which I still contend. My role in HIV medicine allowed me a first-hand look at the horror of the infection and the possibility of creeping dementia and random sudden death. To contest my own doctors' judgment and stay in practice would have been unconscionable in light of the responsibility I had for my patients' care and safety. It was devastating to realize (after my departure from Lawrence Medical Group) that I'd never again be walking through the door of my office and seeing patients—my beloved brothers, the children of Hamelin. I've had to surrender much of my identity as a physician and create anew from that which remains.

The advent of AIDS produced not just the waste of lives, as if anything more could matter, but also this loss of my profession—and with it a measure of my identity. These days I am most often aware of the forfeiture of my career when an acquaintance or friend discusses his or her symptoms, or a disease of some friend or relative, with didactic analysis of which symptom correlates with which disease (some people right, some wrong)—all showing that they have no awareness that I myself, standing there, am a physician. My training and experience are lost; my identity is mislaid.

Our identity may be constituted of little more than collections of choices, habits of emotion and residue of memories, but we can always attempt to override our psychological anatomy and see ourselves objectively. Years of study and sacrifice have helped shape me. But I don't regret this period, for I chose this road myself and others would have dearly loved the opportunities I've had. After all, I've had the supreme honor of being allowed to provide care for many of my brothers before they were taken from us—and for that I am deeply grateful.

SUNDAY ESCAPES TO THE GETTY

For the last year and a half of his life, Jack and I drove to the Malibu Getty Museum for lunch most Sundays which was my day off. Reservations were required and, whether or not Jack was well enough to go, I booked a visit every Sunday. The Getty Villa is a duplication of a Roman nobleman's house, complete with enclosed patios with fountains and benches surrounded by extravagant depictions of Romans at work and play. From the acanthus leaves (signifying enduring life) in the wall decorations to the museum's most prized *Irises* by Van Gogh, Jack and I drank it all in. We would concentrate on just one room of the museum or quietly sit in one of its patios. At the museum we didn't need to talk, we just enjoyed each other's presence. This quiet reflection was all followed by a leisurely lunch outside in the sun under a latticework of vines and flowers. Jack and I spent many relaxing Sundays in those surroundings enjoyed by the aristocracy of ancient Rome.

We had discovered this relatively unknown jewel of Los Angeles long before his diagnosis of lymphoma—and we enjoyed it long after. On our last trip to the Getty, he had lost much of his hair and his weight had deteriorated, his cheeks were sunken, his skin tawny beyond natural. To his credit, he didn't complain during his decline. When he had enjoyed what he had the energy for, he merely asked "Why don't we go?" With each visit, more and more slowly, we'd walk back down to the car together and head home for the remainder of a sleepy Sunday.

LINGERING REGRETS

In the beginning, Jack was able to maintain a matter-of-factness about his malignancy. But as his illness progressed and it became clear chemotherapy was ineffective, grief overcame him and tangled his emotions. During his last months, facing his inevitable death, I sometimes became a target of his frustration. Anger at caregivers is common, I have seen couples break up when the patient had only a few months to live (or sudden romances begun with equally abbreviated life spans). While I am sadly familiar with the phenomenon, the sting was hard to take.

About three months before he died, Jack overheard my end of a telephone conversation which upset him tremendously. I had been downstairs in the kitchen while he lay in bed upstairs. I can no longer remember with whom I was speaking, but the question came up concerning how long he was expected to live. "A few months," I replied with a remote, professional matter-of-factness behind which I would occasionally hide. Unfortunately Jack overheard my half of the conversation and was bowled over by what he heard to be the definitive prognosis and, in addition, he interpreted my remarks as a wish rather than a report. When I saw his agony, I tried to convince him that my statement had nothing to do with desire, but the prediction was more difficult to discount. I told him that I happily imagined his presence with me long into the future. But by that time the fatigue and pain he felt, the tedium of sickness, the frustrated wishes of a life un-lived—all of these caused his emotions to implode into an uncharacteristic paranoia. My remarks left him despairing and bitter and my efforts in explanation, sadly, fell flat and disbelieved. He remained angry with me, on and off, until he passed away. This was to be a great sorrow of my life, that during his last few months there was tension between us. But perhaps his reaction to this overheard phone call was a sign that his illness had finally bested him. If so, I cannot blame him.

JACK'S RIGHT TO LAST RITES

Throughout the years of my practice, I submerged my personal spiritual beliefs in order to provide the most support possible for my patients. Part of my work was to protect each individual's own personal faith, without exhibiting a zeal for their beliefs which would have looked as phony as it would have been. Had I had such believer's consolation, my life and work would have been easier. But my upbringing in the church has inoculated me, as it were, from religion: religious belief, it seems, can't be organic in me. Even if my patient's near-death experience wasn't due to undiscovered human communication and signals from a dying brain, an afterlife seems implausible. In any case, this is a cognitive dissonance I can't resolve. All those in my care deserved whatever religious attention they desired; if I could not provide it, I would facilitate their getting it elsewhere. Jack was to receive no less.

For as long as I knew him, he had never attended Mass. Nevertheless, he considered himself a Catholic—not devout perhaps, but certainly within the Church. His Catholicism seemed to be more a piece of identity, a place for him in a social construct, rather than a rigid set of beliefs. Not being Catholic, the Evangelical teachings of my youth had always held this type of religious expression to be heretical. But regardless of doctrine he lived a life entirely consistent with a belief in God.

When we made that vacation to Europe in the fall of 1989, not knowing his reaction but wanting to be supportive, I floated the idea of visiting the Vatican and perhaps be in attendance at an appearance of the Pope. Would he see healing, or at least comfort, in the earthly embodiment of his faith? The first time I broached the topic, he paused a while before answering. Finally he said yes, but he spoke without great enthusiasm. Lourdes, it occurred to me suddenly, might be something he'd appreciate more and, who knew?, perhaps it would better kindle a hope—hope, our most necessary of currencies—if not for healing, then for something else less tangible. But he had no desire to make the journey to Lourdes. I searched for a papal schedule. This was Jack's life, after all, and I wasn't going to discourage him from any metaphysical comfort. Once we were in Rome, he became more interested in attending a papal display of whatever sort. As I suspected, he wasn't expecting any kind of cure, he only came searching for some bits of hope or comfort which I felt even he couldn't define. But during our stay, contrary to his published schedule, Pope John Paul II stayed at his summer residence and didn't give any Vatican benedictions. Without a word of complaint or discouragement, Jack quietly settled for a papal medallion keychain and a resin angel which he hung above his bedpost at home.

Later, when his illness had progressed, I wrote my father asking for any Bible verses he could give that would be comforting and I could share with Jack. My father, with his vast knowledge of the Bible, could surely provide us with some moving pieces to console Jack, a spiritual Catholic, in his last few weeks. My father, however, sent me "The 4 Spiritual Laws" Evangelical tract—a booklet used to convert non-believers. It was far from the warm and supporting scripture I had hoped. I didn't show it to Jack; I didn't think he needed another medallion keychain.

During his last hospitalization in May, 1991, it was clear he was not going to live much longer. I was distraught, unsure of what to say, what to do. Sickened by his cancer, his breathing became progressively labored. There came a moment, an hour, when it appeared that he was failing. Not knowing what "Extreme Unction" or "Last Rites" actually involved, but believing it an integral part of Catholicism, I was going to do all I could for Jack to participate in it while he was sufficiently aware. He wanted it—that was all that was necessary. Not knowing who would step off the earth first, we had made a commitment to support each other as best we could. His hour of death may have been uncertain, but he had chosen this sacrament of the Church, and to be cognizant during it.

That afternoon at UCLA Hospital, I called the hospital chaplain and requested "Extreme Unction" (also known as the "Sacrament of the Sick" and therefore not limited to those who are dying). After some three hours, a priest was found. I had started the process before Jack's mother Viv returned from a break because I knew, for whatever reason, she would be in opposition. Once she learned of my efforts to procure a priest, she was livid—she demanded the ceremony be stopped. Perhaps it wasn't my decision she resented, perhaps she believed he would be shaken if he knew we thought he was failing. That was possibly true, although I found it an unsettling testament to her faith that she believed the "Sacrament of the Sick" would be more demoralizing than comforting. Subsequent research has shown, however, that a patient's understanding of his or her illness doesn't rob them of hope and calm but, besides providing these essential elements, decreases terror, worry and depression. It also gives him and his family and loved ones time to prepare emotionally and logistically for what is to come. In any case Jack had been adamant that he would receive all of the Church's rites. Viv could storm into the room and throw her opinions and orders around, but she could not countermand his choices made in quieter moments. If he wanted "Extreme Unction" I would see he got it.

He received this sacrament and was, as I had hoped, conscious enough to participate. But he did live to go home once more and I saw that Viv felt vindicated. My mind was numb, my emotions raw. It is impossible for me to say what I felt during those hours between his hospital discharge and his death. I am sure triumph was not the only sentiment Viv had and perhaps I misread her. But this is how it appeared.

DURABLE HOPE

Jack died in the living room of our condominium, in front of the wet bar, in a hospital bed we had rented the week before. Three days prior, he had been discharged from the UCLA Medical Center with hospice care being our only option. The day before he died, in a raspy voice which was hardly more than a whisper, he asked what would be done next—not what could be done, but what would be done. Even hours before his death, Jack, like all of us, needed hope. I told him a fantasy, cloaked in medical jargon, of some remaining treatment. There was still hope, I lied.

But many others were like him; they weren't ready to be told that death was near. Don, the hard-working attorney, on his Friday hospital admission, told me he needed to return to work Monday. His 6'1" frame weighed no more than 100 pounds when I told him that we would do our best. As always, I was to take my cues from the patient, for there is no right way or wrong way to die. This time it was my Jack. If someone wasn't ready for death, it wasn't my place to drag them, kicking and screaming, to a point of accepting something which they couldn't.

Ominously, he had stopped clucking altogether.

I stayed with him on and off through those nights, sometimes sleeping upstairs in our bedroom but usually napping with my head on his bed. I wandered outside from time to time to watch the ripples on the pool outside our door. I've never been a smoker, but I wished I had been in order to gain whatever smokers gain. I wanted him to live forever, and I wanted him to die in the next hour. I wanted him back the way he had always been. Anticipatory grief, that missing someone before they're gone, I now experienced as missing the Jack

I had known before. The playful rascal. The insecure chef. The party planner. The old Jack.

It was in the morning hours of June 4, 1991, when Jack finally passed away, at the age of 43. Over the course of those eight months after his lymphoma diagnosis he had lost 30 pounds and his sparkling smile, but not his will to live. He never gave up and in that there is its own triumph. Denial on the part of one who is dying, or his loved ones, may well impede a tranquility that acceptance would supply, but there is something to be said for a durable hope, for an optimism in the face of constant deterioration and accelerating loss.

Over those last weeks with Jack, I had a recurrent image, a mirage, that lingered on the edge of my consciousness, and which reflected the last steps of the journey we made together. In the daydream I am carrying a sleeping Jack in my arms. He is quiet and peaceful, no longer in pain or fear, and I am able to carry him easily—his weight is not a burden. This half-dream gave me a strange and difficult-to-describe solace.

JACK'S DEATH

During those dark days of chemotherapy, after he had lost too much hair and too many pounds, we found ourselves sitting in a little Orange Julius in a nearby shopping mall. It was there that Jack asked if I wouldn't on occasion wear his ring. To this day it pains me deeply to think he needed to ask for something that was to happen naturally and with reverence. I told him absolutely yes, and there before me, as he sat gaunt and grey-colored, I saw again the smile I had seen on his face those years back in Venice.

There are few things I remember clearly from that morning he died but the most vivid memory I have is of my quickly taking off his precious ring after his breathing stopped and his eyes glazed. Before it was lost or, more likely, confiscated by his mother. Viv had done an inventory of our house during the preceding week and it was clear she intended to take everything she could: everything that Jack owned before he met me, everything we acquired together and anything else she could. And if, in her espionage, she couldn't ascertain what was mine and what was ours, she wouldn't be splitting hairs; if in doubt, I knew, she intended to take what she could carry. The moments immediately after he passed, my objective was uncomplicated—through my tears I slipped the ring off his fourth finger and put it on my own. Jack would get his wish: I would wear his ring, our ring, and he would be remembered, and cherished in that remembrance.

When the two EMT men arrived to take his body away, they asked me if I wouldn't rather step out of the room while they placed him in the body-bag. I said no, I wasn't going to leave him. I sat while they put on plastic gloves and gingerly lifted his corpse, still warm, from the bed and placed his still form in the large black bag and zipped it shut. As is part of our humanity, we feel there is still a part of the person we knew in their remains. For so there is. We honor those bodies of the ones we love. We carefully bury them or, in acknowledgement and farewell, burn them. We visit their graves. It was only when the EMT men insisted that I not ride along to the mortuary, that it was against their rules, it was only then that I acquiesced and let his body go.

JACK'S FUNERAL AND
THE BRUTAL AFTERMATH

Our office manager Pam came to my rescue. She began calling those who needed to know and she arranged for a funeral Mass in a nearby Catholic church. Although I had anticipated dealing with the funeral home, I was grateful when Pam began the planning for me. During Jack's last hospitalization, he was so close to death that I had asked him whether he preferred cremation or burial and, if internment, where. When we first moved to Los Angeles, we had gone on a light-hearted tour of celebrities' grave sites. The sinking realization of what we both faced, however, soon twisted the tour into something more grim than when begun. But neither of us had had anything definitive to say on our burial preference. Later at that far more consequential time I had asked where would he like to be buried. "Well, where are *you* going to be buried?" he asked. "I don't know, Jack, but whatever may happen in my life, even if I might have another relationship, I will be buried with you."

In the end he couldn't decide; he was just too sick to choose a location for his grave. Looking back, I am troubled by my persistence that day—in spite of our previous discussions, I was asking too much of him. The time for such decisions had passed. After all legally I was little more than a roommate. Viv and Gus stepped into the vacuum and over Pam's objections and my peripheral input—domestic partnership, let alone marriage, was not even a possibility at that time—the funeral home gave his parents sole control of his burial. Without discussion or debate, Jack was buried in Collinsville, Illinois. Had it been another time, or had I been another man, I would have demanded I be included in, if not directing, the planning. But I had neither instructions from Jack nor the energy to battle his parents.

Viv vociferously fought against any ceremony—either a funeral or a memorial—in California or back in Illinois. He had insisted that there be no viewing of his body, but he had definitely wanted a funeral Mass. She was beginning to chip away at what I knew he had wanted. There were many, many who had known this wonderful, sweet man and they deserved the opportunity to honor him, to say goodbye at some type of service. I overruled her: there would be a Mass. If there were to be a Mass, she declared, then at least there were to be no flowers. I was shocked—Jack had been a sometime florist! No, I insisted, there were going to be flowers. If there were to be flowers, she persisted, then there was to be no music. What? Was she kidding? Flowers and music at a funeral or memorial service were so universal that it was absurd to oppose them. I was dumbstruck! If she had her way there would be no Mass, no flowers, no music! She disliked me intensely and that could be sufficient fuel for disagreement but it seems unbelievable she would reject or minimize any formal ceremony just to prove superior power. It seemed like it was partially due to a problem with Jack—perhaps it was anger, perhaps shame with him for his sexual orientation—I can only speculate as to her motives. Powered or not by her challenge from me or her disgust with Jack, I found her remonstrations to be absurd and heartless. This painfully showed me just how far issues of power and control can hijack common tradition and common sense.

Now I fought her, not as a powerless roommate but as his spouse. There would be all three—a Mass, music and flowers. I was determined. My plans and resolve, however, thwarted her into full fury.

"Let's get on with it. I just want to get him into the ground as fast as possible so I can get on with my life."

How could anyone feel that way about playful, loving Jack? How could anyone say that? I was stunned to the core. Sadly, Viv's attitude was not hers alone. Years before a mother had asked me, while her 23-year-old son lay dying in the Intensive Care Unit, exactly when he would die because she needed to get back East for work. That mother had said the same thing as Viv: "Just get him buried."

MY EPIDEMIC

173

Viv and Gus ignored the physical care and emotional support Jack received from me; this was the attitude of many families toward the partners and boyfriends who provided such loving care during those dark days. We caregivers often worked alone and without acknowledgment or gratitude. The months I cared for him, I had changed soiled sheets, run for a bedpan, searched for that one food he liked and might eat. I had spent time taking him to doctors' appointments, sitting with him during chemotherapy and those small hours of the night when the terror of approaching death demanded alliance and understanding. This had been my choice but it had been enormously exhausting. Like so many of my brothers, I made the sacrifice of complete submersion in the life of a dying man to the neglect of my own. But once Jack was gone, once our brothers had passed, we caregivers were frequently left with no notice of our efforts and no one to share our loss.

The funeral Mass was conducted in a Catholic church not far from where we lived, by a priest who had never known him. Although the priest forgot to call me up to the podium for my eulogy—a poem of mine that had written itself—the organist remembered my only song request, John Lennon's "Imagine." Outside the church the sunlight was blinding. I don't know if Gus and Viv were there; I have no memory of them. The Soehlke's and I did not grieve together.

I didn't mind as Viv and Gus began taking items from the house. I noticed absent-mindedly that they evidently had no plans for taking the furniture—for which I was glad. The condo and its furnishings, I thought, were some of the few things that still tied me to Jack. However my mind pivoted—many ancient civilizations took the deceased's earthly possessions and either buried them, or burned them, along with the body. Jack was gone. Did it matter what physical expressions remained? Like the remnants in New York apartments, what would one do with these things? They couldn't be protected forever. Suddenly, it seemed, removing many of his contributions to our life was not as awful as it first appeared. Now it hardly mattered what they took—I would have his memory. During this pillaging of the house, standing in the kitchen I nevertheless mentioned some item I wanted to keep.

Viv turned on me. "Don't you get it? You dumb son of a bitch!" Back in our office there was much free-floating anger, but an unbreakable rule of the practice was that no one was allowed to call the staff or doctors names.

ANDREW M. FAULK, M.D.

"Why are you alive? Why are you still alive when you gave it to him? Answer me that, big AIDS doctor, *why are you still alive when he's dead?*"

My mind collapsed as my body stiffened. She was wrong on so many levels. In fact I myself was facing no other end than that of my brothers, no different from that of my beloved Jack. After all, I was another son of Hamelin. I might have explained that her assumption was technically impossible. Jack had never been tested for HIV and without significant treatment available, it was not something I pressured him to do. Our sex life had always been conducted carefully. But the only thing I said was "That's not what happened. It didn't happen that way."

For the first time in many years, I wept. It all came out, the sobbing, the tears. Bleary-eyed I looked down at the kitchen counter and in that moment, for me, the entirety of Jack focused: his charm, his caring, his gentleness, his spirit. I didn't care that Viv saw me crying; I didn't care that she might interpret my tears as some kind of admission of guilt. Apparently the honesty in my voice and my tears communicated more than my lack of explanation.

"Well, if you didn't do it, one of you did. One of you sick perverts."

So it was finally out in the open, the reason for all the anger, all the obstruction and bitterness I had always felt from her. Yes, I had seen disinterest in so many families for the caregivers. But this was different from the usual apathy. Viv had been angry since the day I met her and now she voiced her rage and turned it on me.

Another man might have defended himself, defended us, but that day I had no stomach for it. I said nothing further. I climbed the stairs to our bedroom and walked into our bathroom. Now tears overwhelmed me. All around me was evidence of Jack, from the brightly-colored towels to the funny knickknacks on the counter. It was all him. I cupped cold water into my hands to dunk my face. I looked up and saw myself in the mirror, water running off my nose and hair, tears blurring my vision. My face was puffy, my eyes red, my nose running. I brought my hands up to cover my face to bring some relief, some atavistic comfort, with the touch of my own hands. I wanted to tell her that we didn't know when he was infected, no one knew in those years when we had no evidence until it was too late.

But rebellion, not apology, began to well in me. Viv had called my brothers and me perverts, but love and sacrifice can never be perverse. After all the care, all the love we had demonstrated toward our sick and dying brothers, if some people thought us subhuman, let them think so, we weren't ashamed. No longer hiding in shadow, we were standing in the light. The epidemic had furthered what the Stonewall riot had begun—the destruction of our generation had both outed us and revealed our humanity. The cost was, and is, far too much and I would not have chosen this, our epidemic. But we had purchased with our lives the right to claim our humanity, and turn shame against those who would shame us.

But I did not go down and tell Viv this. In the end, I left what I had said alone. Saying more would accomplish nothing; it wouldn't change Viv's hostility, or accusation, or anguish. At the last, she allowed a graveside ceremony back in Collinsville. Under the awning at the cemetery, I sat in the front row with his biological family. But my position was due to the largesse of the Soehlke family, not my prerogative. I sat where I sat because Jack's family wished it so, not because it was Jack's wish.

PART 2
AFTER PRACTICE

SAYING GOODBYE

Almost everyone has a relationship or two that they would like to change before they pass away. Sometimes I was able to play a small part in mending broken relationships. However, more than that, I could connect with my patients by listening. I could battle isolation of the soul.

The most important thing anyone can build with another person, whether dealing with a terminal illness or not, is connection. In certain situations, only physical presence is possible. It alone is powerful and is the most important thing we can offer. But often we can step further than this.

Although it may be awkward and distressing, tender or terrifying, talking with our dying offers opportunities to achieve intimacy and closure. After our loved one has passed, there can be tremendous comfort in knowing that we extended ourselves beyond our usual boundaries and reticence.

Often, because of the circumstance, we are facing someone who also wants to have a meaningful conversation. They may be as uncomfortable or unsure as much as we are. If it is difficult to begin, it can be helpful for us to ask a question or two which can signal that we are open to listening. An open-ended question, one that's answer isn't "yes" or "no," is the most fruitful. The next step is to truly listen, or engage in what some researchers have called empathic listening. Often our minds are cluttered with matters of our own world and a first step is to quiet our own internal dialogue and devote our complete attention to the other person.

My patients sometimes brought up happy memories or thoughts. Other times, they would show bitterness and hostility. Either way, I found listening from my heart was best. While listening, we must be willing to hear cries for help. If this is what we hear, we may be tempted to jump in and attempt to fix the problem. This may seem to be our role here, but it is my experience that, more often than not, trying to fix a problem is not usually best.

My goal was always to look past simple words and see the whole person. Sometimes, people are too broken for us to engage. If this is the case, we must pay special attention to the limits of our abilities and intuition. It may be best at this point to be still and do nothing. Pushing where there is no possibility of movement will not end well. Surrender in this case does not mean you have failed. I have seen such conversations eventually result in patients reaching a connection with us later, when later is a possibility, or with someone else entirely. We do not always know what good we do.

After listening carefully we can begin sharing our own experiences, thoughts, and observations. These moments can be especially lovely when they are highlighted with humor. However, we need to be careful—interjecting ourselves can be tricky because we don't want to focus the discussion on ourselves; the patient is the priority.

Many will find it difficult to engage in this way, or believe it is beyond our abilities to keep from becoming the center of conversation—if so, there isn't necessarily shame in this, but it is crucial that we know ourselves well enough to understand these limitations and not position ourselves where we cannot help.

I am humbled and grateful for the many who have studied communication with the dying more comprehensively. I do not intend for the following notes to be a complete appraisal of effective communication with our dying, but merely what I have learned by experience and observation during the years of my practice. I have learned that there are several specific phrases that may be used to help achieve clarity and closure with friends and loved ones who are dying. These are:

1. I love you.
2. Please forgive me for whatever disappointment or offense I have caused (even if you believe the dying person was at fault—it is only your ego, not your life. You will thank yourself later.)

3. I forgive you for the disappointments or offenses you have caused.
4. Thank you for your part in my life.
5. I will miss you.
6. Perhaps I will review with the dying person some important, or maybe not so important, fun or funny, shared event, situation or person.
7. Goodbye.

* * *

There are certain types of communication that one may find helpful to avoid. In this situation, these often sabotage end-of-life communication.

1. Don't say "I know what you're going through." Don't compare a situation of yours with theirs.
2. Don't interrupt. Be comfortable with silence.
3. Don't try to fix anything.
4. Don't minimize their situation, pain or feelings.

Scrupulously avoid remarks that begin with "I know what you're going through…" The truth is that no one can truly know what another person is experiencing. Following this remark with any other thought that leads to comparing your situation with theirs will damage your attempt to connect. Such remarks communicate to the individual that your interests are being put above theirs, or equal to theirs, and that they need to convince the listener of their greater suffering.

In so doing, the conversation has been refocused elsewhere and may never recover. After my brother's death in a motorcycle accident, one woman approached my mother and said, "I know what you're going through. My son moved to the East Coast." My mother never forgot this self-involvement, nor the sting it delivered.

Secondly, don't interrupt. Interrupting may signal your centrality to this conversation rather than a focus on them. We must be comfortable with silence.

Too often I've seen people, uncomfortable with silence, jump in and damage the interaction. Let the person speak and, even if it is difficult to judge whether they are finished, side on the air of quiet. For sometimes if we give the other person more silence, more time, other issues may come to light. The individual may introduce another point or brave some other territory. Remember, it's *their* time that is limited.

Thirdly, it is not necessary for you to have answers. People need to be heard. By listening, you are giving this person something they need more than answers—what a gift! Try not to be a fixer, concentrating on correcting things can focus attention away from the person.

My fourth point is that downplaying their symptoms or prognosis is not helpful. Once again, are we trying to make ourselves feel better or are we trying to make them feel better? If we focus on minimizing their grief, it turns attention away from their truth and towards a lie. It isn't possible to build a connection on a false narrative. We may destroy the precious few remaining moments together.

* * *

While my own personal HIV diagnosis was unspoken, I always felt its silent presence and it magnified my ability to connect. In their triumph or despair, I could stand where my patients stood. And I have no doubt that the people I served could feel this resonance While I couldn't provide a cure, I could be fully present and devote myself to listening. Merely listening is profound participation. It is a magnificent gift which both the visitor and the visited may deeply appreciate.

ANDREW M. FAULK, M.D.

A HIGH PRICE

When Jack left us, I made a decision that I would never again have a serious relationship with anyone: HIV-positive or HIV-negative. For me, I could have no second Jack, nor would I be someone else's Jack. To be with someone HIV-negative was inconceivable. Whether or not I myself would need eight months of chemotherapy, one thing seemed certain—the day would come when I'd be in a hospital bed in some living room or hospice. Would someone who loved me refuse to leave the room as they zipped the body bag closed? Would some other grieving man be told it was "against policy" for someone to ride along in the ambulance to the mortuary?

I had been fortunate to have him as long as I did—he had enriched my life and along the way he had created so many trip-wires of memory:

I will never put clothes in a drying machine without his voice in my ear telling me to clean the lint trap every time I use a dryer.

I never load a dishwasher without hearing his howls of laughter the day I mistakenly used *regular* dish soap and flooded the kitchen with bubbles.

Each Christmas I remember the gifts unexpectedly presented to me by his family in Collinsville, and whom I thanked profusely, only to discover later that they had all, in fact, come from him.

My life is immeasurably richer for the memory of Jack quietly handing me a can of soda when I returned from closing the eyes of another one of our brothers. I had known someone who'd stare across a pillow and tell me of the beauty of a soul struggling with my work. And that I was loved. But our relationship had used every ounce of me—I couldn't do it again. I had loved him and the cost had been tremendous. I could not be there for someone else's end; I would not allow someone to be there for mine.

THE SEARCH FOR THE RING

After the 1994 Northridge earthquake, when graffiti began to appear within the walls of my condominium complex, I bought a two-bedroom house tucked inside the Hollywood Hills. In spite of a multitude of neighbors nearby, I looked out the glass wall of my living room and saw only forest. My upstairs had a second bedroom just off the kitchen and it was in this room one day, while watching TV, I took Jack's ring off my finger. (It is a nervous habit of mine that I take a ring off my finger and absent-mindedly play with it). It slipped out of my hand and fell; I bent to pick it up and, to my surprise, it wasn't on the floor. Looking underneath the bed, I found it wasn't there. Not on the bedspread, not in the sheets. My fears escalated as my search widened. Had it rolled into the adjacent guest bathroom? Had it bounced into the sink or bathtub? No. Was it on the windowsill? No. Where could it possibly be? My search was to be repeated in its entirety over the ensuing weeks, and even months. It was not possible, but the ring was lost. Jack's ring, the ring I had promised to wear in his memory, was gone.

In the ensuing months I not only searched for the ring but went to extremes I would not have imagined. One night in a gay bar I bumped into a semi-famous medium. I am firm in my beliefs: I do not believe in hocus-pocus. Nor, in spite of whatever phenomenon may have happened with my patient with a near-death experience, communication from beyond the grave. But perhaps it was possible, I suddenly imagined, that by some miracle he could divine the location of the ring. I found myself telling this "clairvoyant" the story of Jack and me, the lost ring and my promise. The answer from the Great Beyond was less than helpful—the medium reported that he didn't work for individual clients anymore. I felt my cheeks redden. I had embarrassed myself for nothing.

Years later, in 1999, I was in the process of moving back to San Francisco when, as the moving truck was full and I made my last walk-through of the house, lightning struck. There, in the center of my one-car garage, was the gold ring, diamond sparkling, unobscured by any debris or rubbish. It was unharmed, undamaged—the same ring I had placed on Jack's finger so many years ago in Venice. The ring I had promised Jack that I would occasionally wear. One might imagine that I then took the ring and that it never leaves my finger. But the truth is, while I always know where it is, I only wear it from time to time. For the ring, like all these memories of Jack, my medical training in Seattle and San Francisco, my practice with Lawrence Medical Group, and the 50 patients and friends I walked with to the edge—all these memories have a place in my heart that will never be lost. I have AIDS, which is really just a reminder I carry closely the mortality we all share. A reminder to enjoy every minute and press those around me to do the same. To live in a spirit of gratitude. To make every moment as happy as possible. I don't wear Jack's ring every day, just as I don't ponder these memories every day, nor reach my goals for happiness every day. But I have an aim, an ambition, to always live seeing the beauty in the world and in the people I love. To lend my ear and my experiences to those who might desire them, and to be forgiving and gentle with those around me, and myself. And face ahead, not behind.

I BECOME A PAINFUL REMINDER

Having left my practice and therefore having the free time, I went to the 1993 White Party (a huge dance event) held every Easter in Palm Springs. There is a perplexing phenomenon, occurring in both heterosexual and homosexual circles, in which a person appears more attractive when they are with someone rather than alone. Of course with this understanding rides the conundrum that one is available when one is without the date that provides the added allure. After Jack's death, I traveled to Palm Springs in the hope that my availability would trump my solitude. In the end, it was neither of the two physics that kept me holed up in my hotel room for most of the weekend.

Unfortunately there is an unearned shame with nearly every disease, and with AIDS, predictably, it is worse. With fears and prejudices revolving around HIV everywhere, to run into a patient by chance required finesse—the physician's oath of doctor-patient confidentiality was always in effect. As anyone I greeted might be taken for one of my patients with AIDS, it was necessary for me to be acknowledged first. So it was with these parameters in mind that I attended that year's White Party.

I recognized three patients, separately, among the 3,000 or so attendees that weekend in Palm Springs, or rather three partners of deceased patients. Each was with a friend or a new partner. As protocol required, I studiously awaited signs of recognition from each of them. As each noticed me, it was with a little surprise and some sadness that I detected reservation. They greeted me, but each was visibly uncomfortable. The care that their partners had received from me and LMG had been good and I had developed positive relationships with all three, but I found in these survivors a common reluctance to spend any time with me. I could see it in their eyes; it wasn't that they were concerned they would be taken as AIDS patients, rather it was that my presence reminded them of the difficult and painful episodes they had experienced with their loved ones. And they didn't want to be reminded. They didn't want to be taken back to those dark, brutal times of ER visits at 3:00 a.m., hospital nurses attempting IV lines on worn-out veins, battles with families and insurance companies to keep their loved one comfortable and themselves sane. All in order to ultimately wake up one day exhausted and alone. I had been more than a doctor; I had been their supporter, advocate, champion, and their friend. I had been with them each step, but it had been a dark journey. I understood how the pain of these times made them resistant to being around me. Perhaps there was a part of me that also dreaded their presence.

Our memories were too fresh. Our hearts too bruised.

DARREN CLARK
ANOTHER GOODBYE PARTY

After Jack's death I lived in a haze of loss and anxiety which, as painful as it was, had been superseded by the more formidable fog of HIV encephalopathy. If I had had any doubts about giving up my career, they were laid to rest then. I had free time, but it weighed heavily on me as my own demise seemed close at hand. Without the advent of the "cocktail," there was little to be done other than taking what medications we had at the time and keeping my doctor appointments: the life of a "civilian." But thankfully, after a period of almost constant awareness, I lived my life as if I had nothing physically wrong—even when a symptom or two would contest this denial.

Meanwhile life had changed for me. I no longer worked 10 to 12 hours a day. I had enough money—but what use did I have for a savings account?

I bought a set of dining room chairs that were reproductions of those designed by my favorite designer, Charles Rennie Mackintosh. Using his original specifications, an Italian company made reproductions that were beautiful in their design and simplicity. In West Hollywood there is a large complex that houses leading interior design stores and it was in one of several box-like buildings, the "Blue Building," that I found Darren Clark manning the store which sold my chairs. He was in his mid-20s, slender and with a disarming smile and self-effacing demeanor—with just the occasional camp to let you know which team he played on. He moved with the ease and casual grace that seemed to come naturally to his generation, a generation which seemed to have largely escaped the internal and external homophobia which made coming out for some of us so crazy-making.

I was of the generation that came of age when Darren's openness would have been dangerous to career, social standing and living situation—if not physical safety. For we were mistrusted by a federal government which, until 1975, fired us from our jobs for our orientation. I attended Georgetown University's School of Foreign Service for my freshman year in anticipation of a career in the US State Department. As my education broadened and I realized that particular professional choice would banish me to a precarious closet for the rest of my life, I gave it up in favor of law or medicine. For we were largely either mistrusted or disliked by the surrounding society which proffered no empathy or protection. Hollywood usually painted us in devious or menacing roles or as outrageous public personalities limited to "glass closets," such as Charles Nelson Reilly and Rip Taylor. Rarely did we stumble upon the courageous transitional figures such as James Baldwin, John Rechy or Allen Ginsberg. Or hear of the pre-Stonewall revolutionaries Harry Hay or Franklin Kameny who showed us that identity-based movements arise when the state and society insist that one's identity disqualifies them from legal and cultural citizenship.

Darren Clark, on the other hand, grew up in a world transitioning into one largely free of the hysteria and harsh judgments of the old. One of the things I love about California is the comfortable and matter-of-fact attitude with which society accepts us—sometimes grudgingly, but accepting all the same. For the Golden State led the changing national *zeitgeist*: it was surprising and refreshing, albeit disconcerting in its novelty, to swim in a sea rapidly changing in temperature and current.

After studying the different Mackintosh chairs available, I returned a third time to Darren's showroom. He invited me to his back office where we had a coke as he filled out the required forms and I wrote a check. During the three months it took to have the chairs manufactured, he changed from a healthy-looking man, although thin, to one emaciated and gray. Upon hearing that I was an AIDS doctor, he questioned me regarding the quality of care his own physician was providing. I assured him that his doctor was more than capable. The disease was so little understood, the field so new, that when questioned about the quality of other doctors, I only expressed doubts when someone limited their care to Chinese herbs, acupuncture, chiropractic or when there was enough information to label the provider a quack. When my chairs were eventually delivered, Darren invited me back to his office for a celebratory coke.

His disease had progressed rapidly. He had lost weight he couldn't afford to lose. His face now showed the typical seborrheic dermatitis and the all-too-common bi-temporal wasting and the bronzed skin of adrenal insufficiency. Jack's death had left me stunned with little emotion and little to say and I was not asked to offer any false hope—Darren knew his future. Fortunately for my own nerves, he spoke easily, at first about a memory of camping with his late father and then about his own approaching death. He had decided to have a Goodbye Party; he had several credit cards with a significant amount of available credit and had already rented a "presidential" suite at a hotel in West Hollywood. He was inviting his friends to the farewell. Although these farewells ended with what appeared to be the person drifting off "to sleep," I couldn't help but see these grim get-togethers as barely-disguised violence.

I've experienced several kinds of Goodbye Parties—each very different from the others and having its own individual anxiety and desolation. This one seemed to lack the underlying sad desperation of the others I'd attended. The hotel suite Darren chose was very large with a bedroom, sitting room and huge bathroom. Darren loved flowers and there were so many bouquets and "falls" that one might have thought the death had already occurred. Initially there was no cannabis smoking as it was a non-smoking room in a non-smoking hotel. Although it was a day for breaking the rules, the gravity of the event made the participants oddly careful at first. Later they relaxed the rules and their tensions as they opened the windows and smoked both tobacco and cannabis. We obtained some visual relief from the handsome bartenders who seemed, at least at first, unaware of the true nature of the event. Darren had hired a group of five men to sing who were wonderfully upbeat and campy. Their songs dealt, as one might think, with the difficulties of our orientation. Although they were the most cheerful people in the room, they had to have known the purpose of the event.

I went to the hotel alone and didn't spend more than 20 minutes with Darren. I used the excuse that my M.D. license would be in jeopardy should I stay while he took the medication. I don't know whether Darren believed me but he certainly went along with the premise. He had already taken something and his speech had begun to slur and his eyes were slightly glazed. On each side of him sat a friend he had chosen to be with him when he took the final dose. It seemed almost out of place but I told Darren, as I had stressed with my own patients who had chosen this route, that should he have a change of mind at any point, 911 could be dialed and medical personnel could interrupt the effect of the medications. (Obviously I didn't mention the nasogastric stomach pumping.) "Don't worry about it, Dr. Faulk, I'm okay with this," he understated. He had never called me "Dr. Faulk" before.

Although Darren was not my patient, I felt the impact of this Goodbye Party, as I did all of them, to my core. Since Jack's death I cry easily. He had not yet passed, but that afternoon was an exception. Alone in the hotel bathroom, with my forehead pressed against the cold, ceramic wall, I wept. Crying seems to focus and distill free-floating sorrow as nothing else can—perhaps that's why we often feel better after the tears have come. When I left the hotel suite that afternoon, however, the "party" had left me deeply shaken.

ANDREW M. FAULK, M.D.

I AVOID MAIL

When I was still in practice, Jack and I were friends with the couple John Swenson, my patient, and his partner Michael Taylor. Jack and I had been invited to their house for dinner during the Christmas season of 1990. It is another gathering in which I share the memory with only one other person—Michael. John and he had been wonderfully supportive with delivered meals and drop-in visits when Jack was dying, but within five months of Jack's passing, John, too, was dead. His mother had been one of those parents who continued a relationship with their fallen son's partner and the two of them threw a memorial gathering that first Christmas after he passed away. I was invited but mostly I stood alone, speaking a little with only those few who knew me and felt comfortable around my silence. In any case, Michael and I lost contact after that.

Eight years later in 1999, when I moved back to San Francisco with then-partner Lance, I stumbled upon a letter from Michael dated sometime during the period 1991 through 1993 when the years after Jack's death and before the cocktail were the most foggy. The letter, sadly, had never been opened. I am ashamed to say that Michael's letter was mostly about my inaccessibility. He was angry—we had been friends, he thought, and I had become unreachable.

Obviously a great deal of patient care depends upon availability. While I was in practice I was almost constantly available—if I weren't, an on-call physician was always available—but I preferred to deal with my patients' issues myself. However the confluence of my own illness, grief at Jack's passing and the loss of my medical career was an emotional cataclysm to which I reacted by withdrawing from much of the world. Except for the easily discernible bills, I would go weeks without opening mail. A letter could mean news of another death or it could be a request, something which I'd need to act upon. I told myself that I would tackle the mail in a few days, when I was feeling emotionally stronger. I couldn't stand the contact, the shared memories. I wasn't of great difference from the partners of my patients at Palm Springs' White Parties who couldn't stand the memories I evoked.

Whether it was ground mail, email or phone, I avoided communication with all the energy of an obsessive-compulsive disorder. Similar to PTSD in its effect, this fear, no matter how irrational, follows me to this day. No matter the inconvenience and potential for catastrophe, I prefer sending letters and postcards instead of engaging in phone calls and email because this one-way communication seemingly protects me from the possibility of bad news. News that someone else I love has stepped off the earth.

ANDREW M. FAULK, M.D.

JOHN EMBRY
FESTIVAL OF CAMP AND
BEDROCK OF SUPPORT

John Embry was a loud, funny, over-the-top patient who was always a festival of camp and a source of heart-felt assistance to the men he accompanied into my office. His caring was as tangible as his presence. He would often stand with a hand on each hip in the fashion of a wronged drag queen. He had come from Texas, but his chivalry and Texan dialect were the only things left, apparently, of the prudery and convention which surely had been his upbringing. His cultured choice of words made him extraordinarily entertaining and immediately identified him as a son of the South—although in his case more of a disorderly step-child than a bonafide offspring. He punned incessantly, almost always in the direction of the sordid and lascivious and had that *joie de vivre* which comes from knowing one's *vivre* may disappear any day. I must have met him the first week I worked at LMG and, when I initially walked into that exam room in Los Angeles, he was laughing loudly while the assistant took his vitals. When we were alone, he gleefully asked me if I had been "warned" about him by the other docs. I had not been forewarned, but his statement had the quality of a challenge I was not going to let slide. "No, but what would they have said, John?"

"That I'm a loud queer, that I have a lot of friends and that my jewelry is spectacular!"

He hoped to dumbfound me. During the first few months of my practice at LMG, I usually went to work wearing a tie which, together with my thin frame, thick head of hair and glasses, gave me a somewhat bookish, naïve appearance which was misleading.

Intrigued but noncommittal I said, "Oh, is that right?"

He was grinning from ear to ear. "You want to see them, Doc?"

"Of course," I responded.

At that point he unzipped his jeans, took down his shorts, and showed me what he was obviously proud of—and indeed should have been. Along the midline of the underside of his penis was a neat row of eight to ten small, short rods all neatly arranged equidistant apart (a "frenum ladder").

I was the new doctor in the office and John was testing my squeamish meter. But the gleam of the tiny balls on each side of every stud, so neat and orderly, had me. Whatever he may have anticipated I was going to say, I could tell he was disappointed with my response. "How do you get through security at the airport, John?"

Without missing a beat, he answered, "I ask them if I can take my pants off."

"And do they ask you to take your pants off?"

"Nope, Doc, unfortunately they never do."

My unruffled demeanor simultaneously dissatisfied him and provoked his interest. At the time piercings and tattoos appealed more to the "wild child" in me than my appearance may have suggested, but I didn't want to be identified outside of the "geek" classification I had come to encourage. I preferred to fly underneath the radar. I still do.

But John had attributes far more beguiling than his penile accoutrements: he didn't judge anyone who didn't judge him and he was a bedrock of support for many of our patients. Although I may not have been outwardly moved by his unconventional ornamentation, he won my quiet admiration by occasionally sitting in on his friend's medical appointments with them—and sometimes even attending office visits with people he barely knew. He provided a remarkable comedic presence at their various tests and hospitalizations. To many, some as equally perforated as himself, he gave physical and emotional support to which they had little access. To those who were newly facing the sobering kitchen blender of medical jargon and laboratory metrics, his presence and ribald jokes gave enormous comfort and battled crushing anxiety. He was a rock for these men and I soon understood that he was well up to the task of walking my brothers into the emotional abyss of their HIV infection and, indeed, off the edge of the world. In many, many cases, I knew if John were in the room I could move on to those who had no support.

Our friendship grew and soon I knew him well enough to visit him at home. He had lost a substantial number of friends—at their bedsides I imagine. In his living room, on break-fronts and tables, shelves and windowsills, one could see photo after photo of smiling men who received his remarkable attention before dying. These photos included three of his deceased partners.

As his jewelry indicated he was more than a little eccentric, managing a stockbroker business from his kitchen. Monitoring the results of the experimental HIV treatments of those he was aware, he would invest for himself and his friends in those pharmaceutical companies producing what appeared to be the anti-HIV candidates most likely to succeed.

In this winter of loss and sorrow which petrified the hearts of so many, mine among them, John's heart beat constant and strong. He didn't just look after patients. He was one of the few patients who inquired after me personally. I saw him on and off through my years at LMG and our mutual affection and presence in the holocaust raging around us kept us connected. As it happened, he was never a guest at our house when Jack was alive, but he made charming and provocative appearances during the few get-togethers I had at the condo after Jack passed away.

DAVID ST. GEORGE
A LAST WISH

Leaving the practice left me a haunted man. I was at a loss—I had surrendered my career, but I wasn't dead and there was still fight left in me. I could still contribute, perhaps not as a physician, but in some other meaningful way. John, well-known for his ability to network, referred me to David St. George, a man living in Albuquerque who was nearing the end of his life. David lived alone and had no one to provide him care or companionship. I knew I wasn't in a position to provide medical care, but I knew I could provide the presence of someone with medical training.

David flew out to Los Angeles to see me and we immediately hit it off. He had been an attorney and was a short, slight figure, with a reserved, quiet manner; he was the exact antithesis of boisterous John Embry. It seemed he had no friends except casual acquaintances and, of course, John.

David was thankful and, more than anything, joyous about my coming to stay with him for a while. He had the same illness as I: AIDS encephalopathy—disorder of the brain caused by HIV and sometimes ending in an Alzheimer's-like picture. It wasn't anything new for me to spend time with someone who had my diagnosis and possibly be confronted with symptoms which I might develop. I knew these possibilities well. There was nothing new to fear.

His house in Albuquerque was spacious and comfortable and when I arrived, I saw his calendar marked "Andrew arrives TODAY!" Once moved in, the time slipped away with tourist visits to Native American villages and nearby Santa Fe. I hadn't been there long when David told me his one last wish: he wanted to see Amsterdam. He was afraid his health wouldn't permit a trip to Europe but this seemed like exactly the reason I was there. There were to be complications—upon returning from a quick trip to L.A. for my passport, I found his encephalopathy had worsened and he was able to walk only with great difficulty. Together we saw his primary M.D. and discussed it there in the office and, as his mentation was nearly unaffected, we decided to go ahead with his dream.

Soon we were packing and on our way, but it was an inauspicious beginning. The trans-Atlantic flight was incredibly difficult because I hadn't made arrangements for us to sit near the toilets. With other passengers staring in disbelief and sympathy, I physically carried David, in a "dead man" carry, back and forth to the restroom. It was an experience I hope never to repeat. Nothing could have been sweeter, however, after the horrendous plane trip than the excitement of Amsterdam. This was David's "last hurrah" and so the hotel was first-rate, the restaurants terrific and we soon had tickets to see a famous play then being performed there.

But we hadn't been there long when he developed fevers and a dry cough. I knew the likely diagnosis and quickly took him to a hospital. His chest X-ray showed the typical blanket of snow and he was immediately admitted with the diagnosis of *Pneumocystis* pneumonia. Although I looked over the shoulders of the doctors providing his care, I had little to add or question. Dutch medicine was state-of-the-art and Dutch doctors more than competent. With David hospitalized I soon fell into a pattern in which I would leave the hotel mid-morning and spend the rest of the day with him in the hospital—I saw very little of the Netherlands other than hospital corridors.

Toward the end of his hospitalization, David's sister flew out from Chicago. She was nearly our age, easygoing and fun to be around—she brought a lightness into the hospital room and into the trip. Her presence allowed me to see some of the city, although David was on my mind even when I was exploring and she was with him. She couldn't have shown me more appreciation while we were together there in Amsterdam. After about two weeks of treatment, his pneumonia cleared but his mental status remained clouded and he stayed hospitalized another two weeks. The three of us returned to New Mexico where his sister decided to move in with him. It was while I was unpacking him I came upon a bombshell—there at the bottom of one of his suitcases I found to my perfect consternation a plastic bag filled with cocaine! He had packed on his own before the trip and I hadn't seen it. Customs must have judged his condition too grave for us to be worthy of a thorough search for we had passed inspection in two countries. Here I was, taking charge of our entry papers and luggage when all the while we were carrying with us cocaine and a prison sentence!

With David's sister assuming his care, I returned to L.A. In about 10 days I received a strange call from a confused David asking for my forgiveness—but what did I need to forgive? He was too muddled to say, but it was related to his will. I "forgave" him quickly and our phone conversation ended soon after. I didn't hear anything more from him or his sister so I assumed HIV had taken its course.

A month later I ran into John who let me know David had died within a week of his phone call to me. He had slipped into a coma and drifted off the edge. What surprised me was John's report that, in that last week, I had been removed from his will, which had originally bequeathed me $200,000. I hadn't known I was in his testament—nor had I expected to be. Evidently David's sister had taken advantage of his confusion to persuade him to change his will at the last moment and leave everything to her. John's friend, John Li, had also been removed from the will, but had gone to court, without any success, but discovered the various amounts David's friends were to have received. As I'd extrapolated my T-cell numbers and surmised I'd be dead in a year or two, what did money matter? But I was nonetheless touched that he had thought of me.

The story of wills being changed at the last moment was commonplace. Several of my friends and patients feared their relatives would push them to change their wills when they were incapacitated. It was not an unjustified fear; I was to hear this scenario repeated again and again.

I went on to provide companionship and care for two other men with AIDS living in Los Angeles—Thomas Harrington and Gabriel Hernandez. As before, with David St. George, I moved in with them and, for these men with neither relatives nor close friends, I provided supervision in taking their medications, a helping hand to wash and clean and a calming presence to talk them down when the terrors of the night became too great. Both died within several weeks of my beginning to live with them.

After these codas, my emotions were burnt and it was clear to me, I had done what I could do. I could no longer serve.

DANIEL JAMES
"I HAVE NO REGRETS"

John Embry was more than a friend—through all the fog of grief, I remember he and Linda Gromko attended Jack's funeral. Six months after Jack's death, when I was still living in a twilight of sorrow and near-total isolation, I called him and asked him to meet me somewhere. On the phone I said, "Listen, John, I need to be with people tonight. Could we meet at a bar or something? We don't have to talk about Jack or anybody else that's gone. Just hang out." Really, any environment would have been acceptable, but if we happened to drift into the storm, a man crying in a gay bar during those years wasn't the spectacle it might have been in another place and time.

After Jack was gone and I was no longer in practice, I found myself standing in bars far too much. Although I drank little, the hours wasted, I am afraid, were substantial. On my deathbed, should I complain about lack of time, I need to remind myself that I wasted a lot of time in bars during these years. Just the presence of gay men around me, however, provided an emotional respite and, of course, physical safety.

That night John and I chatted about the superficial things people talk about in bars. Neither of us wanted to discuss a mutual friend's death that had occurred the preceding week. But after some time had passed with no words being exchanged between us, he walked over to the bar, found a writing pad, wrote something down and returned to the psychological safety the bar wall provided. He handed me a slip of paper with the name "Daniel James" and a telephone number. "Call him up" John said, "Dating isn't marriage." I took the piece of paper.

Although Daniel was known as "Bink" to his friends, I could never attach that name to him. He was shorter and younger than I, red-haired and small-boned. His smile confirmed his introversion which nonetheless had enough warmth to make one feel they were noticed and accepted. He had a hearing impairment and wore a hearing aid in his left ear and, if one listened closely, they could hear the slight mispronunciation of those consonants difficult for the hearing-impaired to master. Nevertheless, in a quiet environment he could hear much, if not most, conversation but he also relied on lip reading and, much simplified for me, sign language. In spite of this obstacle we managed together quite well and to my quiet satisfaction he once remarked that none of his previous boyfriends had engaged him in conversation as much as I did. He was a handsome man but in the competitive physicality of late 20th century Los Angeles my insecurities made me worry that my looks were problematically inferior to his. His affection and matter-of-fact acceptance of our difficulty in communication, however, made me believe I was allowed a pass in this respect.

Perhaps because of his hearing impediment he was insightful and quick to identify people's qualities. In general, he had a way of emphasizing the good and minimizing the bad that was often infuriating. The fact that he happened to be red-haired, as I am, aggravated my own internal homophobic prejudice that most gay couples appear to be nearly identical. But never mind. Daniel had had a problematic childhood, I knew, but he didn't speak of his family. To this day I know of no details of his childhood or youth or, for that matter, any relatives. It was as if he had no history before we met. In gay circles such breaks with the past were neither unusual nor outlandish.

When I was in high school, my Evangelical Lutheran church routinely sponsored a summer camp for disabled children, in British Columbia. It was there that I learned some simple sign language and how to spell. Years later my training was enough for uncomplicated conversation and therefore I saw all of LMG's deaf patients. For those many situations in which my vocabulary was insufficient, I was still effective because, after all, one can spell *anything*. But Daniel preferred us not to use sign language in public—he didn't like the visible exhibition of his impairment. So in public he lip-read when he could, and nodded assent when he couldn't. There are hard of hearing people who develop a method of navigating in the world which reinforces a distinctive and secretly disparaging exclusivity, but that was not his way and he was happy to draw others in.

Daniel used to proudly repeat "I have no regrets" as his personal mantra. As he frequently and adamantly stated this axiom, I pondered its meaning—both in my own life and in Dan's. Did he consider all mistakes to be intolerable personality flaws or unforgivable blunders of judgment? Or perhaps the opposite was occurring—maybe he narcissistically saw all negative events as originating outside himself. Contrary to Shakespeare's Cassius, did he absolve himself by concluding that the faults in our lives do, in fact, lie in our stars? On further reflection, I believe this was a choice he had made in which he refused to "punish" himself for anything in his past. He saw no benefit in looking back; perhaps he reasoned that there was enough grief in the present. Or that obsessive rumination produces paralysis—which it certainly can. In my life, however, I've done much learning and growing through mistakes and the regret they engender. Recognition of past errors has been a productive tool for me in building self-awareness and side-stepping future blunders; every experience can have positive value. (In full disclosure, when showering, however, I am particularly vulnerable to disturbingly audible "shame spirals.")[3] When Frank or I consider pushing the "send" button on some text late in the evening, we ask ourselves whether we will regret what we've said in the morning; we specifically use the word "regret" in our analysis. I think Dan saw regret only as crippling sorrow instead of a productive mechanism for steering clear of future mistakes. Shortly after moving to San Francisco, my partner Lance accidentally threw my only suit in the washing machine and it came out perfectly fitted for a hobbit. Instead of apologizing for this rather minor flaw in attention, he was adamant that he was *not* going to "feel bad" or apologize for the misstep. I suspect some of the same narcissistic dynamic was in play there, as with Daniel. Beyond the irritating message that any future suit I might own would live in constant jeopardy, he was telling me that his feelings were more important than mine. For he, too, saw no benefit in feeling remorse for past errors—regret was only unhelpful self-abuse.

In spite of my resistance to getting close to anyone, I remembered John's aphorism about dating not being marriage and enjoyed

Daniel as we began spending more time together. But knowing his HIV status, I admit I kept a certain distance. And over time I began to notice an unattractive inclination that some of my brothers, or anyone, without resources occasionally display—the vigorous and often loud expectation of the best in accommodations as well as finding fault with superlative service. Besides this predilection, Daniel had a manipulative mind-set that didn't shirk from using people and situations to achieve his goals. He principally employed fact-bending and small deceptions, but lies are lies and by paying attention I learned more than he intended: if he'd use a friend, I determined, he'd use me. In hearing matters of dishonor, an attentive listener should only presume he is an exception at his own peril.

The experience of my years taught me that such a character failing could not be adjusted with a simple heart-to-heart conversation. Or many such discussions. Had I allowed myself to become more deeply involved, there would have been non-HIV problems partnering with Daniel. When he developed subtle changes of abdominal lipodystrophy (fat accumulation in the belly) and bitemporal wasting, I ended the relationship definitively. While our break-up was inevitable, the timing was excruciating.

Daniel moved to San Francisco and I didn't—at least not at that time. Making myself unavailable for bad news by mail or telephone, I didn't keep in touch with him, but a mutual friend later told me that Dan had died in the spring of 1995. He spent the last year of his life as an impoverished recluse living in a friend's garage. He didn't live to see his 37th birthday.

NORMAN NASH
CONTROLLING PAIN, I AM ESCORTED OUT

About the time I was breaking up with Daniel I found myself back in touch with my New Jersey friend Norman Nash who, in the 1980s, had also lost his partner of a decade. In the spring of 1993 we went to the third National March on Washington together and there, unfortunately, we had a falling-out. He disapproved of a couple of new acquaintances I had made and destroyed their business cards. He had become too protective of me, smothering me in the process, and I ended up withdrawing from him. We hadn't had an argument, I simply drifted away. This is a regret in my life because it robbed me of that last bit of time I could have enjoyed with him. It was a sad miscalculation because it was that September that Norman called. His T-cells had been dropping, he said, and he'd begun to lose weight. He called to say he was dying. My first words were, "No you're not." I tried to quiet him; I told him he was overreacting. While my training and experience may have agreed with him, I simply didn't want to face his death. Another person close to me couldn't die. I spoke to make myself feel better, not Norman. It is a common phenomenon: many people who discourage the ill from frankly discussing their disease have similar motives. They want to ease their own pain. Here I was no different.

"No," he replied, "I'm having constant diarrhea." I can no longer remember my words, I must have told him to have it evaluated. A few weeks later, I got a call from George Jones, his best friend, telling me that Norman was hospitalized in a community hospital near his home in Elizabeth, New Jersey. He was not thought to survive long. I flew to New York.

Norman was in a near-coma state, but his grimaces, moans and spikes in heart rate and blood pressure let us know he was suffering. He had perianal herpes, which causes bone-wrenching pain. There was no way I was going to let my buddy experience this degree of agony, especially when we have good tools for treatment. I went to the nurses' station and, ethical or not, amongst the diligent hyperactivity of the nurses and physicians, I found Norman's chart and read his medication orders. He was limited to Tylenol. No doubt out of concern that stronger pain control might suppress his blood pressure and respiration to the point his life would be threatened, his doctor was under-treating his pain. It is a common, unfortunate misjudgment of a doctor not taking a patient's probable life-span into account when treating pain. I telephoned his attending physician and gave her my best "come-let-us-reason-together" tone. Annoyed that her care was being questioned, she nevertheless agreed to take several of my suggestions under advisement—but after this discussion Norman's pain medications didn't change. Seeing him in such needless agony hour after hour, I first requested that his private doctor be called by the nursing staff and then, in succession, his nurse and then the charge nurse responsible for the unit he was on.

Time passed without intervention. His attending didn't come to examine him and I asked the staff to once again call her. Perhaps they called, but at this point the entire staff was annoyed with me. I didn't care. Who was I, they asked, a member of the family? "No, not exactly, but a good friend who is a physician," I replied. I was angry in my impotence, however. It was obvious to me Norman wasn't receiving optimum care, especially when it came to pain management. He'd fallen victim to inadequate pain control: pain isn't sufficiently treated for fear the treatment might result in either narcotic addiction—irrelevant in these situations—or the death of the patient due to respiratory and/or cardiac arrest. The first is a destructive overlap of medical ignorance and the dictatorial politics of Puritanical conceit and the second is lack of a broad overview of the patient's pain in light of his or her probable lifespan.

It was about 3:00 p.m. when a pain order finally came in from his doctor. We waited while the hospital pharmacy filled the prescription and the nurse piggy-backed the clear fluid into his IV. A morphine drip usually signifies "palliative care"—care to treat nothing more than pain. Norman had just turned 47 and it is difficult for any physician to place someone on comfort care—especially at such a relatively young age. But it was a time when, for many young men, men much younger than Norman, palliative care was the only option.

Often when a patient must make a medical decision which is beyond their scope of education or intuition, it may be easiest, and best, to ask the physician what choice he or she would make if it were them, or their parent, or their child. This can be a welcome shortcut through a forest of statistics and probabilities, a chance to avoid worry and deadly second-guessing. Although it may be our decision, we must trust the doctor just the same. But when our patient can no longer make such decisions, we must earn the trust they gave us in better times. It was a gift I could give him now. He had placed his trust in me and I would prove faithful. He would walk to the edge and beyond without pain or terror.

Comfort care is care.

Once the morphine drip had begun, a great calm descended on Norman: his thrashing and moaning ended. I had had the privilege of providing him, this close friend, the benefit of my years of training and experience—and helping resolve some of his pain.

It was about 3:30 p.m. I looked out of Norman's window down at the hospital's entrance. It was late October; it hadn't snowed yet but it was bitterly cold just the same. Norman was in a twilight state of near consciousness, principally because of the morphine for which I'd fought so hard. His eyes were closed. Suddenly from the hospital bed, he began to speak slowly, but clearly, "The Lord is my Shepherd, I shall not want. He makes me lie down in green pastures. He leads me beside still waters. He restores my soul. He leads me in paths of righteousness for His name's sake..." Startled, George and I looked at him, looked at each other, and then looked back at Norman. Although Jewish, he had never been a religious man. I knew the 23rd Psalm from years of church and Bible camp, and he recited it in its entirety. We were stunned. Over the years, he had generously paid for his nieces to attend Jewish camp in the summers, but that would have had nothing to do with his recitation of the Psalm—especially in English. We weren't prepared for this.

By then the disease had taken a heavy toll on his body. He looked gaunt and frail, with eyes shrunk into their orbits and arms so thin they appeared as if merely shaking his hand might break bones. In this disease one might expect that, with the tremendous transformation of bodies, voices might similarly be affected. A surprising phenomenon, however, was how little damage the voices of those with end-stage AIDS underwent, staying as deep and vibrant as before their illness. A person's physical presence may change beyond recognition, it seems, but their voice remains unaltered. Norman's recitation had been in his usual deep voice that we knew so well.

I watched Norman in that hospital bed; finally, with pain medication, he was quietly sleeping. Suddenly, it seemed, it was 6:00 p.m. and two security guards appeared at the door of Norman's room. They each had questions and *guns*. Was I a relative? I turned toward Norman's friend George who gave me a surprised look. "No," I said, "I'm a close personal friend who happens to be an AIDS physician." One of the security officers placed a hand on his hip and with a dark look in his eyes said, "Visiting hours are over and you're not a relative. It's time for you to leave the hospital." He had said "hospital" and not "room." Evidently my thoughts on Norman's care hadn't been entirely appreciated. I walked between the two security guards to the elevator, through the lobby and out the front door. I guess they thought the presence of firearms was necessary to give me sufficient motivation to leave.

I had been with Norman two days in that last week of his life, and I'd been successful in easing his pain. Norman died the day after my birthday.

THE COCKTAIL AND ME

I lived to see the advent of the miracle-working antiretroviral "cocktail" (two or more medications—three in my case) which became the norm after 1995. This scientific achievement marked an incredible turning point for those with HIV. Before combination antiretroviral therapy, my T-cells (CD4 cells) had been fluctuating in the fairly healthy 350 to 750 range and since the new medications began there has been no change in my counts. My HIV "viral burden," another indicator of HIV suppression, has also been undetectable. Before, in the late 1980s, I tracked my T-cells and extrapolated their decline: in 1989 I was preparing myself to die in 1993 or 1994. But my counts never fell below 350 and, as they never dropped below 200, what gives me my diagnosis of AIDS are my symptoms. After 1996, highly active antiretroviral therapy (HAART), the "cocktail," kept my T-cells in this elevated range which sustained my general health, amplified my cognition and almost certainly increased my lifespan. It is a testament to these new medications that, more than thirty years later, I am still alive.

Since needing to leave my practice, I've been most pained by my impaired cognition—that is, my thinking, memory and learning—due to HIV encephalopathy. But since 2001, I have slowly begun to improve. This is a surprising development, nearly unheard of in HIV medicine, and almost certainly due to the advancement in medications. Because of the characteristic limitations of the brain, and the aggressive nature of the virus, this is one of the most remarkable aspects of my story.

Parenthetically, I also attribute the pronounced improvement in my thinking, in part, to being placed on amphetamine combinations (e.g., Adderall).

Despite the cocktail, however, I frequently encounter episodes of diarrhea which are exasperating in their unpredictability and may be due to HIV or the medications or a combination of both. I have tremors and balance issues which sometimes look like a form of Parkinson's Disease which, like the diarrhea, may be related to HIV or the medications or the two in conjunction. One cannot gauge, however, how these symptoms may have evolved had I not been on the cocktail.

The experience of losing more than 50 patients and friends, along with years of perpetual vulnerability, has left me with some degree of Post Traumatic Stress Disorder. PTSD is well known to cause, among other things, major depression and social withdrawal. As part of this I often feel alone and isolated around others because my life has been singed with death more than most, and doesn't easily mesh with those around me. Dr. Greg Pauxtis has remarked that those of us who were practicing at the time permanently carry a certain sadness because we all live with a cemetery in our minds— "we were too young to have buried too many who were too young." During my practice, of course, my shadowed imagination registered the possibility—the probability—of my becoming, sometime in the unkind future, every patient I examined. These are, and were, not trivial fears. But this element of my PTSD has thankfully decreased over time—I've become better able to remember rather than relive. Expressive writing, in remembering rather than ruminating, also helps control PTSD.

The beginning of HAART was a tremendous breakthrough which leaves me, and everyone living with HIV, incredibly better off. The life-saving cocktail of medications has increased longevity and given us healthier years. In fact these days most people with AIDS die from causes other than those strictly associated with the virus. But CD4 counts above 200 don't necessarily protect one from HIV's accelerated aging and increased cardiovascular (heart attack, stroke) and metabolic diseases (diabetes and lipodystrophy). These complications are probably due to antiretroviral medications or possibly their interface with the virus. The accelerated aging which those with HIV encounter probably decreases our life expectancy by approx. 10 to 15 years. Greater than the statistics our ages would suggest, HIV-positive people are more susceptible to strokes and heart attacks. The metabolic disease of diabetes—both the onset and severity—is statistically higher than in the general population. Besides diabetes, people with HIV occasionally are subject to the disfiguring condition of lipodystrophy—fat in the face, arms and legs decrease while it accumulates in the abdomen ("Crix belly"[4]) and behind the neck ("buffalo hump"). It is a great irony of the disease that the vaunted, ultra-masculine appearance of gym-going men with powerful arms, muscular chests and flattened belly morphs into the far different one of thin arms and legs, scrawny chests and distended abdomens. A fat buildup in the neck can occasionally interfere with breathing and require surgery. There is, of course, greater incidence of these disorders as we HIV-positive men age. I myself have dealt with some of these. Although the cocktail has enabled me to live an unexpectedly long time, none of us live forever. I also realize the longer I live the more susceptible I become to having my uneven mentation deteriorate into AIDS dementia. For me the effect of the cocktail is that the pool may be less deep, but I am still treading water.

Clearly I am well-educated in the last stages of this illness. When it comes to others deciding whether or not to prolong my life, my medical power of attorney is instructed to continue my care as long as I am capable of enjoying life. But discussions about ending care usually occur in a fog of ambiguity and should I no longer wish to eat I ask that I not be force-fed and not treated should a life-threatening infection or condition occur. While obviously not opposed to physician-assisted euthanasia, I find the decision and preparation for the endeavor emotionally overwhelming and I suspect I will allow inertia to make the decision.

Whether living with little hope, as before the anti-HIV cocktail, or much hope, as now, my emotional outlook has remained fairly consistent; as I've mentioned, I largely ignore my AIDS diagnosis but religiously take my medications. For someone less schooled in HIV, an elevated and stable T-cell count, together with an undetectable viral burden, would be ample reassurance. In the small hours of the night, though—when life can seem the most bleak—I struggle with the paradox of knowing too much in a world in which information is usually empowerment. Even while experiencing some HIV-related problems, however, even while taking medications throughout the day, I don't live in an awareness that these intrusions are due to an ongoing illness. However, I did not always live in such nonchalant composure: in the first half of the 1990s, every tickle in my throat was *Pneumocystis*, every flat skin discoloration was KS. My fears were so eccentric and compartmentalized that they're difficult to describe now: an AIDS death was inevitable and, as I was doing the little that could be done, worry and fear were pointless. What I did fear was the inevitable pain of the disease and procedures, the gut-wrenching side-effects of medications, the loss of control of my own body as hospitalizations and clinic visits burned up my time and attention. I feared the pain that would come before death.

But things couldn't be any more different now and I barely remember those days. In fact, I now resist dealing with any problem that's not obviously serious until after I've had it for at least two weeks. Oddly enough this doesn't seem to be as difficult as one might imagine; the emotional costs are small compared to the happiness I enjoy remaining on the planet. They are merely the "cost of doing business." Crucially, I am not married to my illness.

LANCE NEWMAN
THE LAZARUS SYNDROME

Lance Newman entered my life by way of an improbable blind date. In those days between 1995 and 1998, I spent an inordinate amount of time in bars attempting to escape the shadows and whispers filling my head. One night in the early spring of 1998, as I was standing alone in a Silverlake bar, I was approached by an exuberant, heavy man with red hair and a beard to match, introducing himself as David. He "hit on me" and I told him thank you very much, but no, he wasn't my "type." Usually that would be enough to end further discussion but my new acquaintance persisted, "Well then, what's your type?" After pondering the downside of airing such personal information, I told David those preferences I was comfortable giving and we parted.

Weeks later I was in the same bar when David surfaced. "Listen, I've got a guy for you." Having forgotten our earlier conversation, I couldn't imagine what he was talking about. "You know," he said excitedly, "I found someone who matches your list and whose list matches you! I have his phone number right here!" Yes, a date and I were to be introduced by a perfect stranger who knew almost nothing about either of us.

Lance and I ultimately met in a Los Angeles restaurant and clicked as David and I had not. He was dark, handsome, and my ideal in many ways—a sexy man with intelligence, education and an ease in living in his own skin. Before the advent of the highly active antiretroviral cocktail, Lance had been profoundly ill and, as a matter of fact, continued to suffer painful neuropathy. I was comfortable with him—he understood the struggle with HIV.

For a time, however, I was wracked with worry that I was putting myself at risk for the exhaustion and heartache of walking another partner off the edge of the world—perhaps trauma I might not survive a second time. Eventually though I made the conscious decision to ignore my fears as they were borne of an immutable history and, instead, resuscitate hope and nurture its survival as a counterweight to these terrors. For I realized that when the range of possibilities are considered honestly both safety and jeopardy are illusion. I reasoned that perhaps I could place confidence in myself to withstand the punishing maelstrom of another partner's passing. For whatever strength and resilience I had acquired had been forged in that same furnace as my fears, and thus had in them that same durability.

While I had fully lived the emotional pandemonium of the epidemic, I dreamt of a sustained period of calmer, happier times enjoyed with a partner. I didn't want my relationship with Jack, wonderful as it was, to permanently demarcate the parameters of my life; I wanted my time with him to merely color one piece in a broad spectrum. Whether it was to be an illness of Lance's or an illness of mine, I would make a leap of faith that either would be manageable. And should I be the first to sicken, I would have the experience of someone else pushing my wheelchair, holding a bucket while I retched, cleaning my soiled sheets and washing my bedpan. It would be a shattering lesson in surrender and humility, but hopefully one I would transcend.

In any case, David had struck gold for me; in a matter of weeks strangers were asking how many years Lance and I had been together. In January of 1999, he and I exchanged vows before an attorney and friends, signed domestic partnership papers, and celebrated with the fizz of champagne!

Our relationship grew until we traveled east to Philadelphia to visit an old girlfriend of his. Above her home office desk was a photograph of Lance when he was at his medical worst; I was horrified to see him in the pale, emaciated state of someone with advanced disease. Previously I thought I had come to a point of accepting any exacerbation in his illness, but this photo created an emotional shock which hijacked my thoughts of any future for us. For me our thriving relationship suddenly withered and in the space of a few hours became untenable. In spite of my concordat with hope, I thought I simply couldn't do this again—I couldn't nurse another partner through his passing. After an extremely strained month, however, the beauty of his loving support and companionship calmed my emotions and I began to recognize in him the scope of the "Lazarus Syndrome"—the cocktail-induced nearly miraculous rapid improvement in health of many of those terminally ill. I never told Lance of this crisis, how could I? And when our relationship eventually did end, fear of an impending holocaust of illness and grief didn't play a part. Lance and I had had an extraordinary relationship, but no break-up goes well and ours was no exception. On St. Patrick's Day, 2004, he moved the last of his things out of our apartment. In spite of the wisdom in separating, I was seriously bruised.

But that was years later. Early in our relationship, San Francisco beckoned. I was tired of L.A.'s traffic and constant, oppressive sun and heat; besides, it only rained two or three days per year which I found to be unsettling and depressing. Besides better weather, at the turn of the last century San Francisco was one of the most gay-friendly cities in America. Here, one was presumed to be gay just as often as not. By late 1999 Lance and I were settling down in its famous gay neighborhood, the Castro. I began to sculpt, and then paint with shattered glass on canvas in a style all my own, while he pursued his astrology and, happily for me, cooking. We bought a house on the Russian River in Guerneville. I was happier than I'd been in years.

ANDREW M. FAULK, M.D.

LOUIS BRYAN
DISABILITY DESCENDS

It was about the time when I had just moved back to San Francisco from L.A. when I heard from Louis Bryan, whom I knew from my days as an intern. Louis, who had lost his lover, Allen, more than a decade earlier, had planned a dinner for me and Lance. Louis was a busy man, with many friends and commitments, so our get-together had been scheduled weeks in advance. Yet when Lance and I arrived for dinner, we found him in a state of anguished panic. He had forgotten our dinner entirely and was despondent; he had just returned from the office where he worked and had walked out without notifying his team, or even turning his computer off—at the time, a "dot-com sin." Louis, who as a tech writer translated computerese into English, had been experiencing more and more difficulty performing his work, until that very day when he had been overwhelmed by its complexity and his own failing skills. Beside himself with confusion and despair, Louis was bewildered as to how he could continue such intellectually-demanding work. He was pacing and rubbing his breastbone compulsively and one could easily hear his Texas dialect.

It was clear to Lance and me that, like so many other friends, patients, and, indeed, both of ourselves, his working days were over. To lose such an enormous battle in our struggle against the virus was a crushing, but necessary, realization. Often one's friends played a part in acceptance—Dr. Feraru had done as much for me. I sat Louis down and asked him to concentrate on what I was about to say: "Louis," I said, "this is it for you. All of us reach a point where we can no longer work, and attempting to prolong our occupation only makes the situation worse." Louis' mouth gaped in stunned disbelief. "Think, Louis, how overwhelmed you are now. Stress exacerbates HIV. Think of the pressure you'd avoid if you faced the truth now and gave up your job, because the work you're doing will only get more difficult with time and worsen in quality. You could end up being fired and lose your disability insurance." Louis was aghast. "Your day has come. Work is over for you, Louis, but life isn't." I could see the realization wash over his body like a tidal wave; he knew I was right. Louis didn't cry that day, or even tear up, he just stared blankly at the floor for what seemed an eternity. He looked up, he would give up, he would quit work. But he would not quit living.

To this day Louis remains thankful for our arrival that afternoon. Before that hour it wasn't in his consciousness to give up work. He was struggling with how to function in the face of stumbling concentration and faltering skills, and he was losing the fight. In reaching a point of understanding the necessity for this drastic change, the input of others can quiet the noise. It is easier, of course, to bring another person to that place of loss once you've been there yourself. I could help him see the truth; I had been there myself. In many ways, I still am.

LOST IN A WHISPER

John Embry and I didn't see much of each other, although occasionally we would get together with other friends for dinner. Then I met Lance and he and I made the move to San Francisco. After the move whenever Lance and I visited L.A. we would drop in on John, but I saw him less and less as our trips south became fewer. On one of these trips, however, Lance was occupied and so I called John to go out to the bars with me, like we had done in the past. Soon we were standing around talking small stuff. Neither of us mentioned the many we had known who were now gone. But we were both quiet as I drove John home that night. When we arrived at his apartment, I got out of my car to hug him. As he walked up the little hill to where he lived he spoke without turning around,

"*They're just shells, you know. That's all that's left.*"

Almost certainly he spoke of our bodies—the cocoons we live in now—which are buried or burned when we die. I'll never know his subtleties of reflection as I didn't stop him to ask. That was the last time I saw him.

I hadn't seen John for several years when Hurricane Katrina hit New Orleans in 2005. I saw, as did everyone, the TV reports of the devastation and lack of medical personnel. Although I was rusty, I volunteered to serve with the Red Cross in any capacity except as a physician. I thought I could be of service even if just a body far from the "glamorous" epicenter of New Orleans—in Dallas, say, or Atlanta. I truthfully told them I had AIDS and, to ensure I was a help and not an unplanned hinderance, my star of a partner (not yet husband), Frank, offered to pay for the travel and hotel costs, as well as accompany me to ensure I remained healthy. I attended a Red

Cross class for voluntary medical personnel and emailed my plans to a short list of people close to me. John responded immediately with a return message saying the Red Cross would be lucky to have me—even as a rusty medical doctor with AIDS.

The Red Cross, even after their own volunteer training, subsequently turned me down and I licked my wounds. More months than I care to admit passed without John and I communicating. One night I was on the phone with a mutual friend of ours, Bill Litts, when he mentioned in passing John's death. I was surprised, but not shocked, to hear that he had died. When had he passed away? Of what had he died? Bill couldn't help; he didn't know any details. I called another mutual friend, but that friend's phone had been disconnected—another friend gone missing in the age of HIV. I berated myself for not keeping in touch, although it would have been contrary to one of my 'rules of the plague' I had developed by default: you didn't keep in contact with people unless you and they had been extraordinarily close. But John had meant a lot to me—we *had* been extraordinarily close—and my resistance to attachment had been to my painful disadvantage.

He'd been so faithful in holding friends tightly and yet my last visit with him had been rushed and short. In spite of my education and training, it was John who had been the most persuasive in showing me the need, and perhaps strength, in staying close to treasured friends. All the flat surfaces in his house had been crowded with photographs of his friends—many more deceased than living. He had kept a picture of my Jack in his living room and, indeed, had attended his funeral Mass. In these years, protease inhibitors or not, friendships had to be constantly cultivated, bonds had to be maintained. Or they were gone in a moment, lost in a whisper.

MARK HIGGINS, M.D.
"CONDUITS OF HEALING"

Mark Higgins, M.D., my primary physician, spent many years volunteering at the Haight Ashbury Free Clinic in San Francisco. Mark observes that we can't always be "conduits of healing," we can't always be messengers of relief. We may have impossibly high standards that create guilt, but our resources are limited nevertheless and there are times when we must retreat and nurture ourselves. An army can't go to war unless it is fed and clothed. Although I am loath to say it, perhaps this should color our thinking at least a little when we are tempted to judge our brothers on the occasions when we see what appears to be cowardice or desertion. During these times when we see someone who appears to be taking the easy way out, perhaps we should wonder how well their soldiers are fed and their army clothed.

That being said, there are still times when our internal compass tells us that our actions and understanding were deficient. We feel self-reproach for not being there for a loved one in his or her time of need, or for going on to experience years of life after a loved one is gone. These are some of the bruises and lacerations of "survivor's guilt." I wrestle with the regret of not having been a better friend, not having had more patience, not saying aloud what my heart felt— guilt that I wasn't a better person.

There are times when I suddenly suck air into my lungs when stumbling upon a memory, moments when I wonder if my troops could have fought harder, longer, with what they had.

Before pursuing any relationship, even before there was an HIV test, I had considered the possibility of one day walking a partner off the earth. I may not have admitted it—even to myself—but as this was always a hazard, it was always a fear. In San Francisco, I had seen what partners of the dying had paid in chronic despair and bone-crushing exhaustion—the energy spent keeping the spirits up of not only one person but two. And the staggering grief that was the inevitable, the certain, outcome. Once there was a test, I screened potential friends and partners according to their blood serology— their HIV status. While it was always painfully invasive for me to ask this of someone I had recently met, it was vital in constructing a future relationship. Even as little more than a friend, what future responsibilities might fall to me? Years later my physician, Dr. Mark Higgins, told me its name: it is called "sero-sorting." The situation in which one vets their friends and potential partners by their blood serology—their HIV status. Those of us who lived through this period have experienced something rare—on occasion we've felt compelled to let laboratory findings veto relationships.

Many of us have sero-sorted.

FIGHTING GRAVITY

After I left the practice, Fred Lawrence and I spoke infrequently, but on one occasion we discussed the death of one of our patients who was a famous Walt Disney lyricist. He lived in New York, but sometimes flew out to LMG for a second opinion and information on possible new medications. He had passed away just before he had won several national and international awards. Isn't it an incredible shame this man died, I considered aloud, right when all these good things were about to happen for him? Fred responded that, to the contrary, it was a perfect time for him to die—right when the world was at his fingertips, when he was at that exquisite moment when he was anticipating phenomenal success. What a great time to die!

I don't know that I can sign on to this way of thinking.

To this day, when I hear the lyrics of one of his iconic theme songs, no matter who I may be with or where I am, I can't help but tear up.

Sometimes I believe I am wearing internal bifocals: one part frightened by the future, one part, detached, interested in how it will play out. As life moves on, I find that I visualize myself as a fragile space shuttle that shudders more and more intensely as it hurtles towards an explosive rendezvous with the planet. As it encounters the force and friction of the earth's atmosphere, it shakes and tumbles toward destruction. Frailties in the craft are such that it will not survive re-entering the earth's atmosphere.

Yes, most people with HIV die for reasons other than strictly AIDS. But I am no exception from my brothers who suffer from the accelerated aging that will take those 10 to 15 years from us. In spite of the miraculous anti-retroviral cocktail, as my spacecraft speeds to collision with the earth, I may come into contact with a stroke, heart attack or diabetes. Although I've dodged the "buffalo hump," I haven't quite managed to escape the glancing blows of diabetes and "crix belly." As I age, as my craft plunges towards the earth, I expect these collisions will occur more frequently.

The vehicle of my body endures these increasing forces that predispose me to these complications as the disease progresses. As we are all destined to die, this is admittedly an overly-dramatic and narcissistic picture. In fact all of us are speeding toward earth with gradually increasing velocity and, at any moment, may encounter thousands of dire possibilities.

All that any of us can do is buckle up and cope with the shocks and turbulence as we enjoy the ride. But when the subtractions begin to come in earnest for me—especially when I need to surrender my car keys—it will be a dark day.

ANDREW M. FAULK, M.D.

STAN RIDGE
THE SURVIVING PATIENT

On June 27, 2009, in San Francisco, Dick Bretto had a Pink Saturday get-together with a few guests, one of them being Stan Ridge of Arizona. "Pink Saturdays" are the Saturday evenings before Gay Pride Sunday. When I was still in practice in Los Angeles, Stan made the trip from Phoenix every few months to see me. The cornerstone of his personality is calm, measured logic. I don't remember if his status had been discovered with me, but if it had he certainly didn't exhibit histrionics. He's the sort of person who takes such information in stride, acknowledging the natural fear, but quickly moving on to the next step, whatever it may be. In many ways, he reminded me of myself—logic told him what's done is done and the goal was to be happy and fulfilled, despite any possible impending catastrophe.

By the time he walked into my exam room in 1990 more was known, paradoxically, about how little we knew. And with that knowledge came insight into the awful limitations of medicine. We could prescribe AZT, but little else. In a short amount of time, the tools of pentamidine and later septra for PCP prophylaxis would come. But for that particular time it was not only logical, but also oddly calming to concede the limitations of medicine and live daily in that acceptance. As someone living with HIV and knowing I was doing the most I could do, I was free to live life without constant worry. What would happen, would happen. It was an era of making the best of one's time. Stan's visits were matter-of-fact and even serene, especially as his disease wasn't progressing.

At the time, my personal HIV status was not discussed with any of my patients, including Stan. For the questions remained: would a hospital, insurance provider, or senior physician be accountable if an HIV-positive doctor were to disclose the fact? I had found myself out of one closet only to find myself in another. But living quietly, below radar, was second nature. Dr. John Gamble at CPMC had never known my status, saving him the potential storm of lawsuits or cutting me off from patient contact. He may well have suspected the true reason for my attempt to resign, but suspicion was one thing, admission quite another. Neither Fred nor Vincent knew I was HIV-positive, and Stan naturally didn't ask. Long before President Clinton's precipitous armed services policy, physicians with HIV were already living in a "don't ask, don't tell" world.

When I left my practice I told Stan of my disease. So now on Pink Saturday some 25 years later, he and I stood looking down Castro Street from its junction with Market Street, with hundreds of jubilant gay and lesbian revelers. We stood, side by side, our hands resting on each other's hip. "It's so great that we're here, that we both have survived to see this together," he said.

"Yes, it's really incredible," I said as we gave each other a hug.

In my practice I had many patients. I don't know where they all are; I don't know how they all are. But I know of only one patient that survived. He is Stan.

THE MAGIC JOHNSON REACTION

Today is Michael Jackson's funeral, and as I watch Earvin "Magic" Johnson give a eulogy there, I am reminded of when he surrendered his basketball career on November 7, 1991, after announcing he was HIV-positive (after long denying he had "the AIDS disease"). No doubt he made his decision in the belief, shared by so many of us, that his life would soon end. And duplicity in keeping such a secret from a sensationalism-loving public would have been onerous and, in the end, unsuccessful. But the outpouring of acceptance and good will by the general public was met with bitterness by many of my gay brothers—bitterness toward a public which, before a celebrity's mention, had shown so little concern or even acknowledgment of this disease which had felled thousands of us.

After Jack's death, I had begun participating, finally, in an HIV-positive group of healthcare providers. Actually, I only learned the group was made up of those who were HIV-positive themselves the first time I attended. I had signed up on the advice of a colleague for what I thought was merely a group of healthcare professionals working with AIDS patients, not necessarily for providers who were positive themselves. While it was jarring for me to find I was accidentally disclosing my positive HIV status, I was no longer constrained by any potential legal ramifications.

My support group felt not just resentment but outright anger toward this outpouring of sympathy for the celebrity Magic Johnson. The media quickly proclaiming him as "the face of HIV/AIDS" was especially galling.

"Now, suddenly, they've heard of HIV. Now, now that somebody famous and likable has contracted HIV, somebody 'sympathetic,' they see us? How many people have died and they're just discovering us *now*?"

The day after Magic Johnson's death, ACT UP/LA distributed a flyer reporting that nearly 1.5 million Americans had been diagnosed with AIDS before Johnson's disclosure.

DOPPELGÄNGERS OF GRIEF

There were occasions when we children of Hamelin would be someplace—perhaps a grocery store, a restaurant—and out of the corner of an eye we would see the back of someone's head, the side of a face, the tilt of a neck, or a slope in the shoulders. Perhaps it was a familiar tone of voice or a chuckle we had heard a thousand times. A breath would catch in our throat—could it possibly be the lover now passed? Our remembrance would trump the reality; our past would betray the present. Moving closer for a better look, our stomach would drop. No, of course it wasn't him. Our senses were fooling us, tricking us into fantasy. The collision of perception and reason would launch us into accidental heartache and we would quickly look away in equal parts embarrassment and anguish.

Or we would feel someone looking at us—in that same fantastical way of recognition. A stranger's attention snared, we would feel a desperate sidelong glance of disbelief. We'd read a thought as if it were our own: a stranger was seeing someone else in us. This experience was repeated, multiplied, over and over. Gay men got used to certain looks, or the approach of a stranger, because they understood they bore resemblance to the missing. All of us, the children of Hamelin, got used to being mistaken for a loved one.

The awkwardness of such an encounter with a *doppelgänger* of grief sometimes forced an introduction of sorts. But the resemblance was difficult to move beyond and the opened wound would ache the heart anew.

FRANK JERNIGAN
OUR PARTNERSHIP

Frank Jernigan and I began dating in 2004 when he was living in a one-room studio filled with orchids and an elderly cocker spaniel. He was a fascinating man: compassionate, brilliant and, I was eventually to learn, tremendously generous. Frank was unlike anyone I had ever met.

His life had not followed any ordinary trajectory. After being a self-described "Jesus Freak" in Berkeley in the hippie years of 1969 and '70, he married a deeply spiritual woman, Karolyn, with whom he has two daughters. He went on to pastor churches in Maine and Massachusetts and eventually came out to the world—and himself—at the age of 43. Karolyn and he divorced, out of necessity rather than antipathy. But the home-church they helped found was disinclined to choose love and humility over dogma and summarily asked for Frank's resignation. It is the nature and history of our family to be at remarkable peace with each other—thus Karolyn has become a good friend of mine. She is a remarkable woman who, among many things, has a gift for listening to others—especially in an organization for those living on the street. She volunteers for a group that sets up chairs on the city sidewalk to listen to anyone who wants to talk. In 2000, after years studying computer engineering, Frank moved from Boston to San Francisco for the dot-com boom which soon became the dot-com bust. Applying to different computer companies, he was hired by Google at the age of 55—a company at that time famous for the youth of its employees.

It was early in our relationship when Frank invited me to the 2004 Google Christmas party. When he suggested I wear a suit, I

ANDREW M. FAULK, M.D.

took it more seriously than he intended. Neither having one nor the time to buy one new, I descended on my local secondhand outlet with a frenzy borne of desperation. Although I found a suit, it was comically too large and I threw myself on the mercy of an untried, although handy, neighborhood tailor. Having given him as much time as possible, I returned only to discover my suit augmented rather than diminished! With only hours to go, I should have opted for needle, thread, and a few surgeon's knots. Instead, I reached for my stapler. That night I was to discover that staples itch ferociously.

The Google engineers were oblivious to my ongoing discomfort which only entertained Frank the more.

He is now my legal husband—an officially-recognized relationship inconceivable in earlier years. For gay couples multiple anniversaries are not uncommon and, fortunately or unfortunately, they provide opportunities for both celebration and memory failure. We were initially married in our backyard in 2007 and then legally in San Francisco City Hall on November 4, 2008. An historically inauspicious day, that November 4 was the election day when the infamous Proposition 8 passed which suspended further same-sex marriages in California. Like others of that period, however, our marriage remained valid throughout the ensuing legal battles.

One of Frank's daughters, Sadie Valeri, has become an internationally-recognized painter in the classical realism style, while her husband, Nowell, is a pianist, vocalist and extraordinary music composer. Together they had their own art school and now do their teaching on-line. Frank's youngest daughter, Angela, and her husband, Niels, are both Ministers in the United Church of Christ. Angela is a community worker—she strives for changes in racial justice and human belonging; Niels is a healthcare chaplain who works in hospice care. They both are deeply committed to ending racism. Together they have our one grandchild, Leah, who, at age 13, comports herself as if she were 23. With her intelligence and her concern for others, her life trajectory will be awesome! Never having had children, it is quite a shock to find oneself a grandfather!

For the first time in my life I have a long-term relationship with someone without HIV, and Frank has remained so throughout our years together. Having come out later in life, Frank never experienced being a 23-year-old wearing tight jeans and a t-shirt waiting in line outside some club at midnight in the pouring rain. He never was the young, gym-obsessed, fashion-conscious, urban, gay male. Nor has he suffered the brunt of a horrific avalanche of friends and lovers developing AIDS and dying. He has largely lived several degrees removed from HIV and the turbulence it brought to the gay community—which is gratifying and disconcerting at the same time. When I was in the turmoil of my practice, I presumed that life for our society could never, ever be the same—that it never, ever *should* be the same. But Frank's world didn't encounter such heartbreaking, catastrophic upheavals—his has been a different universe. While I more than occasionally feel the solitude of my history and illness, I celebrate his escape. And though he's not very familiar with AIDS, we married when we both knew I had the disease. Many HIV-negative men would have declined such a marriage, knowing the possibility that their husband might well face this savage assassin. Had our positions be reversed, I myself would have thought long and hard and I may well have declined. Instead he opened his heart and allowed our relationship to flourish, and so it has changed my life.

These days his isolation from the disease is no longer what it was. My day-to-day life is punctuated by occasional episodes of what he and I call my "Swiss cheese" memory—unpredictable "holes" in my short-term recollection. I frequently become irritated with Frank for his assuming I remember something I don't or for assuming I don't remember something I do. But how can he predict what I'll recall and what I won't? My memory is not the only thing which makes life perplexing: my diarrhea is occasionally overwhelming, my balance and tremor worrisome. I tire easily and find it exhausting to be around people for long periods of time. But throughout these thorny difficulties Frank has proven himself a loving partner.

NICOLA (CHRIS) BUCCI
FRANK'S VISITS TO SAN QUENTIN

It is Frank's understanding that much happiness comes from improving the lives of others and he works to help those whose help is most needed. Before he retired Frank established a foundation for the advancement of human well-being. Every December we Jernigans assemble to happily choose various groups and individuals to be recipients of the Jernigan Charitable Foundation. While the Foundation's contributions are deeply satisfying, Frank's efforts have not been limited to financial donations. One of his acquaintances, Nicola Bucci, was a chef at Google who was in a terrible car accident that happened without the involvement of alcohol or drugs. In 2008 he was wrongly convicted of Second-Degree Murder and sentenced to 23 years to life; he presently is an inmate in San Quentin State Prison. In our courts witnesses must swear allegiance to truth; it is a shame that District Attorneys aren't required to make the same commitment. "American justice" may not be an oxymoron, but it is hyperbole.

While others have ignored Bucci and his situation, Frank has worked tirelessly for his release. He has contacted the State Attorney General's office, written letters to US Representative Nancy Pelosi and other congress-persons as well as the ACLU. Frank visits Bucci in San Quentin every weekend but, as part of the "hoops" he has to jump through, he must make a pre-visit request two weeks in advance and then, at the prison, wait for an hour and a half and go through two security examinations. Bucci is never far from Frank's mind—we've been in London and he has taken the time to visit people who knew Bucci and perhaps could help with his case. While

Bucci may have been forgotten by his old friends and society at large, he hasn't been forgotten by Frank.

"Spiritual" is a word Frank rarely uses, but he earns it every day just the same.

THE CHAIR UPHOLSTERED IN MEMORIES

We have room on the first floor of our house here in Noe Valley for the things we don't have room for elsewhere. The blending of furniture naturally occurs when a couple moves in together and a rose-colored winged chair of mine finally found a home here on the first level. Last night my eye caught a bit of tag hanging from its bottom carriage that I hadn't seen before, and which had no doubt surfaced in the chaos of cleaning. The tag is the "customer reference" slip showing the chair's date of order as 5/16/91 and its "scheduled ship date" as 6/14/91—10 days after Jack's death.

During that last year of Jack's life there were the usual multiple hospitalizations which accompany the diagnosis of AIDS and cancer, and I was scurrying to find distractions to keep his mind occupied and his spirits up. One of these diversions was ordering this winged chair that now stands as mute reminder of those days. Years before I had sat next to Jack's bed and placing the order for this chair drew our attention away from the surroundings of his room there in UCLA Hospital and became a welcome distraction. Choosing a color and fabric design had helped make it a brighter day. Like the framed posters I hung in his room each hospitalization as a way of giving him something on which to focus, as well as bring something non-institutional into his room. These posters—as bits of our home—were visual reminders of his latest survival. The winged chair, with its comfort of enclosing arms, did the same, if not more.

MY WORST NIGHTMARE

Since being in practice, a particular nightmare has haunted me more than any other. It is not the most frequent, but it is arguably the most disturbing. When I have dreamt it, I have been known to talk in my sleep (unusual for me) and when I awaken I am upset and depressed throughout the next day. When it first began in 1990 I experienced it once a week or so, now I am relieved to have it only about twice a year.

In my dream I am in a darkened warehouse directly beneath one harsh solitary light. Parked askew from each other are two trucks which are nearly identical. I see very little of their cabs, but they're old-fashioned, and their beds, being without roofs, are constructed with wooden sides and wooden floors.

I am pulling long crates, one at a time, from one truck bed and pushing them onto the floor of the other. The movement of these boxes produces a loud scraping sound which breaks a dead silence. My efforts are steady, but the work isn't particularly tiring and the pace is manageable. In the world outside our dreams, I would be unable to perform this task due to the size and weight of these objects. But in dreams, as we know, there are no such limitations. In the first weeks I experienced the dream, I would load and unload them without notice or knowledge of their grim contents—the horrifying awareness of exactly what I was carrying would evolve only gradually. In the years following, by contrast, I have immediately known what these boxes were and my dreadful work.

For they are not simply crates, they are coffins.

And this terrible vision is magnified by the fact they are not ordinary coffins—they are caskets made of glass. I can clearly see into and through all of them. Each one has within it a corpse: a figure which is visible, a body which I can see. Emaciated and horribly disfigured by KS lesions, the cadavers shift and rock from the motion of my work. These are my brothers.

More disturbing than the gruesome setting is my mission. This is the crux of my nightmare—more than the bodies I see is the awareness that I am fundamentally powerless against the juggernaut of AIDS. In the real world I could treat some of the opportunistic illnesses which HIV presents along the way, but in my dream I am merely transferring patients' remains from one location to another—I am rearranging chairs on the deck of the Titanic. I can't affect the slaughter, and this understanding washes over me as forcefully as a tidal wave, sucking my breath away and drowning me in its undertow.

SURVIVOR'S GUILT

Until I die I will face a burden of guilt which cannot be detached from my survival. If I could separate the confusing feelings of grief and guilt I carry, I would be more able to cope with each. But I don't experience them in tidy, discrete packages. Instead I experience swirls of emotions which flow into and out of each other, creating a painful and bewildering maelstrom. Grief is one thing, guilt is quite another, but it can be difficult for me to distinguish where one begins and the other ends. Unless I am vigilant in policing my thoughts with consciousness and logic, the two combine to form a whole bigger than their parts.

The most powerful guilt I feel comes from my survival during a time when those who died and those who didn't seemed monstrously random. I live with the haunting sensation that I should have died along with my brothers. Guilt comes from deserved blame, but here the blame is undeserved. This false culpability, manufactured from the underlying sense that in my survival somehow lies the deaths of my peers, presumes a zero-sum situation—a circumstance in which, should someone live, I die. If I should live, then another dies. Sometimes my self-esteem stumbles and I face accusation arising from the warped perception that many of these deaths are of people I judge to be better than I. Blame cascades onto more blame as I gauge their lives as impacting the world more than my own. Such thinking, of course, is neither logical nor legitimate: my value is as great, of course, as any other. But my guilt from surviving rises and falls from time to time, situation to situation, memory to memory. When a bullet misses you and kills the one standing next to you, are you to blame? What if the one killed next to you is your best friend?

Your lover? I must continually remind myself that there is no fault in survival—the lengthening of my life does not cut another man's short. Although I am innocent of the deaths of those around me, these are feelings, they are emotions, which, in the end, do not easily respond to logic.

Having been a physician during the plague I am also painfully battered at times by the feeling that, if only I had done more for my patients, they would be alive today. These men were in my care. They were my responsibility and they died. How can I not bear some blame for their deaths? Had I sacrificed more, somehow, would fewer of my patients have died? Throughout the day I walk with ghosts and, at 3 a.m., these false feelings of responsibility for their deaths feel monumental.

We now have the anti-viral cocktail and HIV is more manageable, yet I am hounded by the sense that in some parallel universe in which time is inconstant, the medications of today were available in the past but left unused, with terrible consequence. This is not a rational imagining, but I feel it just the same. The truth of that time was that we could treat an infection or condition here and there, but it was a never-ending case of winning the battle and losing the war. Thankfully, today, it is more of a truce.

Yet our only shortcomings were those of medical science, not training or dedication. We did all that we could with the tools that we had. But the residue with which I struggle are emotions which are automatic and reflexive and don't readily respond to arguments of logical reasoning.

There is another type of guilt distinct from that described above, derived from what I did and didn't do in the non-medical realm. When I think of Jack and the many I loved, I can easily bury myself in a blizzard of regrets for those acts I didn't do, efforts I didn't make, and qualities I didn't have. Why didn't I do this or say that? Did I provide all the support I could? Did I fail those near me during what remained of their time on earth? There are times when this blame, this emotion, is the most heavy of them all.

Today as I navigate my course through the eddies of grief and blame, I strive to keep in mind the worth of my brothers and the courage of their struggle without assuming the self-reproach that I, too, should have passed away. I harbor blame for the failures I made with those I loved, but I must forgive myself—for to forgive is to release. And there exists little benefit in holding tightly to the past. Little benefit in allowing feelings greater weight than thought. Living my life as fully as I can and as happily as I am able does not lessen my innocence. Those that have passed away were people whose lives illuminate and inform my own to this day, and I do them no disrespect by living without regret or recrimination.

CONFRONTING DEATH

The prospect of death prompts a philosophical evaluation of life which bleeds into how I comprehend and *feel* about my death.

Sometimes I am able to "accept" my death, at least that's the wording that comes the most easily to me. But it is not my death I struggle with; rather it is the heartache I experience in the anticipation of the all-encompassing loss of myself—the demolition of all those millions of memories and idiosyncrasies, thoughts and feelings, that are unique to me and make up who I am. To paraphrase Clint Eastwood's character in the film *Unforgiven*, "death takes away not only what you have, but everything you'll ever have," while the philosopher Heidegger more precisely describes death as "the impossibility of further possibility." The greater truth that supersedes the glib is that what I battle is not fear of being dead but rather the despair of losing a future.

I don't deal with the anguish of that impending loss as a one-time event, position or even journey. I slip and slide through the Kübler-Ross stages of grief—denial, anger, bargaining, depression and, yes, acceptance. I approach these different plateaus at different times and frequently revisit those with which I have previously struggled. I question myself—am I moving on to another stage or am I revisiting one I thought I had reconciled? It seems I can manage the anguish in one moment and be far from comforted the next. The place where I spend most of my time and energy, however, is in this state of "modified denial": I don't take notice that I have an illness but I swallow my medications and visit my doctors just the same. But even this one form of denial isn't and can't be permanent.

I realize that many whom I envy believe death doesn't result in oblivion but rather eternal companionship and serenity. I know these people enjoy an equanimity which helps them achieve longer and less troubled lives. I wish I had such convictions; but no matter how motivated, a belief in an afterlife doesn't occur organically for me. When I attempt to believe in a God, I have the overpowering feeling I am just fooling myself—as if I were trying to convince myself to believe a placebo was true medicine. I can't embrace philosophies which deny the laws of nature in favor of what is, for me, intellectual anarchy. If I could, my life would be easier. Yet the story of my gentleman who experienced a near-death experience argues in favor of a spiritual world of which I am so skeptical. These two explanations, spiritual and scientific, defy integration, which leaves me stranded with a dramatic and muscular cognitive dissonance.

The existential kernel of death, it seems to me, is transiency. Philosophical Buddhism focuses on the temporary nature of all material things and, indeed, of life itself. When I intellectually grasp this impermanence and feel it, I realize the way to love anyone or experience anything with the greatest depth is to be conscious that all things are passing and destined to be lost. At the end of the film *Blade Runner*, the narrator notes that in the last few moments of the artificial human's life, when the "replicant" poignantly comprehends the fragility of life and his approaching extinction, that is when he loves life the most. When I am aware of the passing nature of life, I am in contact with the passion and depth of living, but also—in that awareness—I can accept the fleeting essence of reality as natural and inevitable.

Jack lacked the surety of eternal life and couldn't acknowledge his coming end; the last day of his life he asked for the details of our future medical strategy. Recognition is necessary for acceptance and as he didn't concede his end he sidestepped a greater battle. Although escaping this struggle, he paid for the evasion by spending valuable energy that produced little resiliency. His partner before me, Ted, was a man I never met. But evidently after the epidemic exploded, Ted became a hypochondriac—his realization of the disease with which he was living produced constant fear that any cough or lesion was the beginning of a death spiral. If anything, stress itself can cause full-blown AIDS to develop more quickly. I knew many men who developed Ted's reaction and spent their remaining weeks in the same emotional chaos—in the end his fears eclipsed his happiness and wasted precious energy.

It is no surprise that my daily struggles with the recognition of my coming extinction produce an awareness of transiency. Viktor Frankl, a Nazi concentration camp survivor, writes "the transitoriness of our existence in no way makes it meaningless... everything hinges upon our realizing the essentially transitory possibilities."[5] Those "transitory possibilities" draw me in to a way to deal with the sorrow of impending death and, surprisingly, provides a route to happiness. I may dislike the phenomenon, but I know by experience and research that happiness doesn't correlate with wealth in achievement or goods. I imagine I'll be happy if I become this or obtain that, but once I've attained this position or acquired that item, my happiness becomes tied to yet another goal or object, and so keeps drifting out of reach. With the comprehension of my impending death, however, the value of the present becomes tangible. And this awareness that all I see and feel, every object and moment, is destined for oblivion makes me love all those bits and pieces of life all the more. I am propelled into loving the present more than fearing the future.

WE SHALL OVERCOME

At the 2009 National Equality March on Washington, D.C., Stan Ridge, a former patient of mine, and Frank and I are introduced to Trudy Shepard, the mother of Matthew Shepard, who was tortured and murdered in Wyoming in 1998.

* * *

In the spring of 1987, there came a time when it was necessary to conference with a family on how aggressive to be with the care of an AIDS patient near death in our ICU. His mother, sister and brother had flown in from the Midwest while our patient, having pulmonary KS, was *in extremis*. He was on a ventilator, in a medically-induced coma, and therefore unable to communicate with us. While we could possibly lengthen his life by a week or two, longer than that was very doubtful and we needed instructions on how aggressively to treat him. The family listened quietly, although the sister fidgeted constantly. She was not in the healthcare field and her questions showed that she was out of her depth. Each time we mentioned one of the possibilities that could lead to patient improvement, the sister became more agitated. Finally the question she had been wanting to ask surfaced: "Can't we do something to hurry his death along?" We were stunned. It fell to Dr. Ron Elkin, the ICU attending physician, to respond and we waited for his answer. Ron was a very low-keyed person but we saw his eyes widen with her question. Before he could reply, she continued that she had flown out to San Francisco leaving her job behind and needed to return by office hours on Monday. She needed to get back to work.

Ron responded that "hurrying things along" was not only legally questionable but ethically unconscionable. She stated matter-of-factly, "Well, you're doctors, aren't you?"

"That isn't what we do," he answered flatly.

She was obviously disappointed with this response. "Well, I have to be back by Monday, you all need to decide what to do," she stood up and walked out of the room. By the following Monday she was indeed back at her job. Her brother had passed.

* * *

David Mixner, civil rights activist and author, spoke at the National March and choked up when he spoke of parents not willing to visit a gay son in the hospital. Once rounding on a sleeping LMG patient, I noticed an opened greeting card standing up on our patient's tray table. I knew little about this particular patient as he was routinely seen by Vincent or Fred. It may have been improper, but I picked up the Hallmark card which on the face was printed something painfully unrealistic about wishing he got well soon. On the inside, across from some printed message equally as vacuous as that on the front, was a handwritten note, "Peter, we know that if you would just repent from your sins, and ask Jesus into your heart, God will heal you. As long as you continue living in sin, though, we don't feel right coming to visit." It was signed "Mother."

Peter died the following week.

* * *

There at the National Equality March on Washington, I looked at the huge crowd and thought, We have all lived with this burden our entire lives. We have been judged, excluded and made to pay a price for the differences in our natural hearts and for escaping suffocating closets. But it is only time before we win our freedoms and rights and, I have no doubt, acceptance. My father already accepts me and has grieved over his past treatment of me—one day America will do the same. This resolute understanding was woven into the fabric of the demonstration and its unifying theme: "We shall overcome."

A SURVIVOR

It has been over 30 years since I was in that exam room receiving the worst news of my life. Although my generation was decimated by AIDS, I have survived the epidemic. The certainty of my imminent death was mistaken, for these days most HIV patients die from something other than AIDS. The medical difficulties I have and many medications I take, as well as the underlying limitations and isolation are significant, but they are manageable. They are, as they say, the "cost of doing business."

There's an old word in German for the advanced education one receives from serious illness: *Siechtumsschulung*. From my long struggle with HIV, I've developed certain goals that, while not necessarily realized, are clear. The most important objective I've found is mindfulness—the awareness of where I am and what I am doing in any given moment. The immutable past and the unknowable future can drain attention away from the most important piece of time we have—the present. Living each moment fully, I've found, can interrupt pointless rumination. When we live in the moment, we're more likely to act in it and more likely to ensure that those we love know they're cherished. Continuing awareness of the possibility of a sudden end doesn't have to mean living in fear of the future, but rather it can serve as powerful motivation to live more fully in the present and with focused attention.

I've learned happiness is an accomplishment more than a condition. Many of my brothers, when pushed to their absolute limit and in incredible distress, chose a road which led to a better place than where they began—a place of giving and forgiving. Living with the possibility of coming pain and loss of control has taught

ANDREW M. FAULK, M.D.

me that happiness can often be found in simple, uncomplicated activities. That it's easier for happiness to occur when I live in a spirit of gratitude. That I can relax knowing that worry burns precious energy, for I can do what I can do and no more.

My work was extraordinarily difficult—not just in intellectual challenge, but also in emotional demand. I discovered, however, a transcendent meaning in work which occurs when we serve a purpose beyond ourselves, for a meaningful life is more satisfying than merely a happy life. My life has been fuller because I was committed to a mission in life: I was going to give my brothers a relationship with their doctor through the long fight they couldn't hope to win. Feeling committed to a meaningful mission in life gives one courage and strength. I believe one of the most important attributes I myself had was not focusing on what couldn't be changed, what couldn't be cured. Rather, focusing my energy on what I could do to help contributed to my resilience. It became apparent to me that we can achieve a consciousness of overriding significance when we focus attention away from ourselves and towards others; there is a unique satisfaction which comes from this redirection.

Resilience is the ability to navigate adversity and to grow and thrive from challenges—redirecting attention away from ourselves to others is just one way to develop and maintain it. Although I didn't know its name at the time, I depended a great deal on the "Stockdale Paradox", named after Vice Adm. James B. Stockdale, who was a long-term prisoner of war in Vietnam. The Paradox holds that surviving adversity means combining both optimism that you will eventually prevail, with a brutal view of your current reality; we hope for an improved future while being honest about where we find ourselves. But we must hold both convictions simultaneously: one without the other only leads to disappointment or despair. I believe that efforts to create outlooks that are not real or realistic aren't helpful; submerging our minds in pretense instead of hope requires significant energy while not giving us the toughness and flexibility we're seeking. A lie requires energy. Resilience depends on a positive outlook, married to an honest reality. A good first step is taking meaningful action. Ask yourself, what's something I can do today, even if it's small; something to remind myself that I am not helpless?

Relationships are critical in maintaining resilience; it's easier to be resilient when you're not struggling with your challenges alone. Although I failed to do this with mental health professionals, I was diligent in creating connections with my patients. I may have seen this as helping my patients, but in fact it helped *me* tremendously. During my medical practice I had Jack, who was invaluable to my equanimity. And, even though they were rarely with me, I knew there were people on this globe who were cheering me on. They may not have been with me at that moment, but I knew they were out there. Although I rarely saw her, Linda Gromko in Seattle was a rock I depended on. This, too, added to my resilience.

Our capacity for resilience is also found in our environment and the systems we live in. For example, such systems as healthcare, mental healthcare, and even more mundane things, such as house cleaning. Our resilience is also affected by our environment and the systems we live in. On a broader scale, having access to a robust healthcare system and proper mental health support can allow us to face challenges with a feeling of safety and security. However, even more mundane things, such as a tidy home or office, can contribute to mental fortitude. No amount of material commodities can be a substitute for having people around you that support you, even with small things like cooking meals. I didn't have mental healthcare, but my access to medical care with Dr. Bill Owen was always available. Since practice, I've learned that resilience can also be more actively developed—but it takes work. One researcher suggests questioning ourselves for every decision we make: does it help or harm? A third glass of wine—help or harm? Going out for a walk—help or harm? Highly resilient people have a strong moral compass. My history of Evangelical Christianity, and the judgements and injuries I've seen and experienced, gave me a strong sense of right and wrong. This, too, added to my resilience.

Siechtumsschulung, if nothing else, has taught me priorities in terms of perception and thought. The British playwright Dennis Potter, dying from pancreatic cancer, wrote "Things are both more trivial than they ever were, and more important than they ever were, and the difference between the trivial and the important doesn't seem to matter. But the nowness of everything is absolutely wondrous." While it's still a challenge to maintain my equilibrium in the face of consequential incidents and accidents, I've discovered it's rarely difficult to deal with the trinkets of disappointment and aggravation

ANDREW M. FAULK, M.D.

we all encounter daily. I am no longer completely invested in a particular result—for example in conversation with Frank, he or I may comment on a desired event or hoped-for result and then one of us will say "or not." We may be passionate about an outcome, but we're also prepared for it to end differently than we'd like.

Having acquired a measure of *Siechtumsschulung*, I hope that when the time comes for my walk off the earth, the courage and serenity of so many of my brothers will surface in me. That I'll reject the poison of self-pity and continue to fight for what is possible in the midst of what is not. Struggle and surrender, intermixed.

I believe that in remembering the bright and the beautiful lost to this, the greatest plague in generations, we not only do them honor but also acknowledge that the work found in helping dying people face their end has its own value—its own success in unsuccessful times. Viktor Frankl writes in *Man's Search for Meaning*, "They must not lose hope but should keep their courage in the certainty that the hopelessness of our struggle did not detract from its dignity and its meaning."[6] When it comes to so many of my friends who have died, I can say I gave the best friendship I was able. And for my patients who, almost to a person, have passed, I rest in certain confidence that I did my best to treat their disease and gently prepare them for approaching death. A quote I treasure says "People may not remember exactly what you did, or what you said, but they will always remember how you made them feel. Remember, what you do echoes in eternity." My hope is that how I made my patients feel will echo throughout eternity.

EPILOGUE
COVID-19, HIV AND
AMERICAN HEALTHCARE

As the speed and scope of Covid-19's destruction shatters our societies, we are developing a visceral understanding of the word "pandemic." Pandemic means people around the world are vulnerable to the same disease at the same time. The phrase "greatest plague in generations," as applied to HIV, is no longer true—HIV has now been eclipsed by the coronavirus. It means that we are all in this place, this place of vulnerability, together. "Pandemic." Its definition enlarges as its impact grows: it means more than it did yesterday, and tomorrow it will mean more than it does today.

Each of us has a definition of the coronavirus. For many of us it means photographs of tearful, exhausted medical workers and pictures of the famous and not-so-famous we have lost. We see bulldozers digging huge burial trenches while statistics of our dead and stories of heroism and tragedy fill our TV screens.

For medical workers, the word will become synonymous with triage. With thousands and thousands of unplanned Emergency Department admissions, triaging will become universal and absolutely necessary. The American medical system, severely limited by political chaos, and a fragmented system of testing laboratories and for-profit hospitals, will force physicians to decide who will live and who will die. In some hospitals there will be, and already are, printed criteria posted on the walls of Emergency Departments: notices detailing which patients have the most chance of surviving, and therefore should receive the most care.

For others, the word has come to have a far more personal definition. Pandemic means hurried goodbyes muffled by white masks and last looks obscured by plastic goggles. It means gurneys carrying away those we love through swinging doors into cold, sterile rooms filled with commotion and bright lights. It means that it is no longer possible to embrace those we have lived with and those we have lived for. It means a stranger behind a face shield asking us how far we will go in a battle that may not be ours to win. It is a crescendo of fevers, sweats, coughing and shortness of breath until our exhausted chests give out and we slip into unconsciousness as we drown. Pandemic can mean dying afraid and alone.

There are those who will define it as the loss of a critical paycheck exactly when budgets cannot stretch any further. It means getting up very early to win a place in the front of miles of cars slowly snaking their way to the food bank outlet. It means waking up in the middle of the night wondering how to pay the rent and which particular credit card bill to pay this month. It can mean calling on a friend or relative for a loan... or a couch. It can mean choosing between hunger and homelessness or disease and death.

Others will define the word in yet another way. We see bars, restaurants and beaches filled with people shoulder-to-shoulder, singing and shouting, without heed of recommendations for masks or physical distancing. They either disregard or disbelieve that their behavior may result in infection or death and they are oblivious to the probability that they may bring the virus home to infect their families. While this population isn't limited to the young, studies show that the highest level of risk-taking occurs in emerging adults (approx. ages 17 through 23) and is more dependent on peer pressure than poor impulse control.[7] It's mostly the young who believe they are indestructible, but there are others subject to willful ignorance and political persuasion. Trump rallies are arranged by people who know the strength of peer pressure very well, and whose goals outweigh the safety of their countrymen. Unfortunately, here the word "pandemic" may become tinged with the regret and guilt generated by careless trips to the beach or rallies without regard for the health of our loved ones nor ourselves.

Eventually we will each gain our own understanding of the word "pandemic."

* * *

In the past we've been unconcerned about pandemics and, if

ANDREW M. FAULK, M.D.

we thought about them at all, relaxed in the conviction that our government would protect us. With the coronavirus this certainty of defense has vanished. *Without vaccine or treatment, there is only one effective protocol for mitigating the disease: widespread testing, contact tracing and strategic quarantines. While face masks, hand washing and physical distancing are critical, they are not enough.* In fact, the number of cases is skyrocketing exponentially while our political leadership is not only paralyzed, but actually broadcasts deception and misdirection. A third of our people are passionately anti-science and argue against even the most minor medical steps, such as mask-wearing, as politically motivated and therefore fraudulent.

One becomes immune by surviving exposure to a disease or vaccination. When most of a population is immune to an infectious agent, this provides indirect protection—or herd immunity—to those who are not immune to the disease. *The number of dead required to develop herd immunity will be a monumental tragedy, and I am not alone in suspecting that, without political leadership, this is the inescapable future for the US.* We are facing the perfect storm of an indifferent and incompetent federal government stumbling around in ignorance and arrogance. Dr. Paul Volberding, an early HIV researcher, judges that HIV will kill, over time, approx. 98% of those infected; the fatality rate of the coronavirus is thought to be in the neighborhood of one percent. (The fatality rate for the typical seasonal flu is 0.1 percent; the H1N1 flu of 1918 is thought to be 2.5-6 percent.) While Covid-19 is more infectious than HIV, both viruses can be spread while the infected is asymptomatic. Yet Covid-19 doesn't always produce illness and has a gestation period of 3 to 14 days, just long enough to profoundly hinder tracing. At present Covid-19 has neither treatment nor vaccine. It is the number one cause of death in the United States and probably the world.

* * *

The coronavirus has killed more Americans than those lost in the wars of Korea, Vietnam, Persian Gulf, Iraq, Afghanistan and 9/11 combined; with our present trajectory we will have lost more than 200,000 by November's election. In the past, our politicians have convinced us of a need to spend billions of dollars on military budgets which balloon yearly. We now see such priorities are tragically flawed—our military expenditures can do nothing to protect us now.

* * *

AIDS is only one of many plagues that the world has faced during the past decades, but it continues to stalk us, and has killed more than 32 million worldwide. But not only do we have treatment, we also have pre-exposure prophylaxis (PrEP) which, taken by someone HIV-negative, protects him or her, by about 98%, from acquiring the disease by having sex with someone HIV-positive. But the great majority of nations have no defense other than abstinence and prophylactics and, even after nearly 40 years, there is still no HIV vaccine. A coronavirus vaccine is much easier to develop than one for HIV: we believe Covid-19 antibodies are effective in attacking infection, we know HIV antibodies are ineffective in fighting HIV. Nevertheless, developing a coronavirus vaccine is not an easy business and it is misguided to depend on one soon.

Our initial inability to obtain broad and rapid testing has been a critical failing. A nation that once produced eight fighter planes an hour during World War II is now incapable of making simple cotton swabs. As initial testing was hamstrung by the CDC's defective testing kits and the FDA's (US Food and Drug Administration) deranged testing restrictions, several commercial labs and universities developed tests of their own. Unfortunately these were not utilized because our fragmented, poorly organized healthcare system made it difficult for hospitals to overcome bureaucratic obstacles. For years large national laboratories have been consolidating their influence by buying up smaller competitors and negotiating exclusive deals with the large hospital chains. The result of this lab centralization has resulted in our nation's limited testing availability and long lag-times for results. Relying largely on two large commercial companies, as we are now, has proved to be a major vulnerability. Relying on these commercial monopolies has been devastating. Despite calls for more than a decade to create a national laboratory system that could oversee a testing response in a public-health crisis, this has never happened.

Our medical system hasn't been able to provide what our nation desperately needed because there hasn't been financial incentive for private companies to stockpile supplies. Although a public-health administration was designed for such pandemics as Covid-19, in the past decade the budgets of local public-health departments shrank by as much as 24%, while private healthcare spending grew by 52%. Today, public-health claims just three cents of every health dollar spent in the country while 97 cents goes to private care: insurance, deductibles and any other costs our health system demands. Meanwhile, the budget for the CDC has remained flat—it is dwarfed by the one for our military which cannot protect our citizens from viral deaths.[8]

Those countries that have done the best controlling the virus have established public-health systems, which quickly developed carefully-planned regimens for testing, contact tracing and strategic quarantines. In spite of the thousands—if not millions—of new jobs this could have created, and its medical necessity, the Trump administration never attempted such a response. As with AIDS, the Covid-19 pandemic has forced the US to recognize what is required of our leaders and our healthcare structure. In his feckless delinquency, however, President Donald Trump has left the nation stranded with only the 14th-century technology of stay-at-home orders. Without leadership and government coordination, there have been devastating shortages of personal protective equipment, testing materials, ventilators and other supplies. The federal government, under Trump, has left states to bid against each other for available supplies—even as federal entities have stolen purchases from hospitals and state governments. Trump's dereliction and blind worship of the free market has been so incredibly radical that he has left our government, and even the union of the 50 states, in tatters.

Other Trump Administration forces are tearing the Union apart as well. Without planning and coordination, different states "opening up" at different times produces infectious hot spots migrating from city to city and state to state. As one state's intensive care units fill because of policy decisions made elsewhere, animosity develops. New York, New Jersey and Connecticut are attempting to quarantine visitors from Florida and elsewhere. Cooperation among states is not just about neighborliness but also about self-interest. So long as interstate travel continues, inadequate testing anywhere threatens public health everywhere—including in places that have found or developed localized testing capacities and are less sensitive to the bottlenecks that LabCorp and Quest are experiencing. The scientific facts are clear: the epidemic cannot be effectively mitigated without a universal, national approach.

To our detriment, the US government is heavily weighted toward the chief executive. Both Ronald Reagan and Donald Trump first responded by denying their respective epidemics existed, then minimizing them, and finally evading responsibility by transferring blame. Reagan never took the trouble to actively deny the existence of AIDS, instead he chose a passive rejection; throughout most of his presidency, he simply ignored the gay community's devastation and the potential reach of the disease. His proposed federal budget for 1986 called for an 11% reduction in AIDS spending: from $95 million in 1985, down to $85.5 million in 1986. Consider that for one year, Mayor Dianne Feinstein's AIDS budget for the City of San Francisco was bigger than President Reagan's AIDS budget for the entire nation. Behind the scenes Reagan argued with his Surgeon General, C. Everett Koop, as to whether it was necessary to even mention the epidemic, let alone assault it. The first statement from the government concerning AIDS didn't come from Reagan himself, but rather was a Press Secretary's answer to a question doubting the President's awareness or interest. Over time, Presidential stand-ins responded with sickening levity which down-played the importance of the disease and redirected attention towards the victims. Press Secretary Larry Speakes conveniently combined two of the classic responses to epidemics: he both minimized its victims and blamed them at the same time. When Reagan eventually remarked on AIDS, it was little more than that—a blip on the screen of national discourse.

The two Presidents handled their respective epidemics in historic parallels: Reagan attacked the character of the individuals infected, Trump minimized the number of those infected. When more in-depth answers were required, Reagan pretended he was interested in combating AIDS; Trump, with his profound intellectual and moral limitations, didn't even attempt to hide his focus on the appearance of the statistics rather than in fighting the coronavirus itself. Their sophistication was of different magnitude, but their approaches were predictable: they assured us that they, and the governments they hid behind, were blameless. Trump's romance with "game changing" cures signaled that he wanted an immediate distraction, rather than

ANDREW M. FAULK, M.D.

actual cure; being a man with the psychological inability to admit guilt or failure, a quick fix would mean the need to concede neither.

Reagan's silence stands in sharp contrast to the unfiltered logorrhea of our present chief executive. However, Trump's earliest responses were also one of denial—first he denied the presence of the disease, then its spread and finally, its importance. His responses to reporters' questions evolved from assurances that the disease would melt away "like a miracle" to emphasizing his personal "success" in minimizing the number of deaths compared to mortality projections. Although the dangers of the virus initially convinced him to discontinue the verbal sepsis of his beloved political rallies, he found solace in hours-long public coronavirus "briefings." His endless ramblings not only failed to convince an American public of his intellect, but instead earned him outright ridicule for suggesting that people should ingest disinfectant and engage in rectal light therapy. Once he brought himself to believe that the pandemic would surely end on its own, he returned to his self-adulation and aggrieved paranoia in assemblies of his most ardent supporters. This placed them in such obvious danger that his campaign demanded signed releases protecting him from legal responsibility for any resultant infections.

After Trump's tactic of bullying governors to "open" their states backfired, he simply lost interest in the national disaster and defaulted to his magical thinking—a pathology based on a breath-taking narcissism which leaves him indifferent to the countless number of American lives lost to Covid-19. In Trump's world, objective reality is subject to his interest and engagement. If he refuses to believe in something, it does not exist. Assessments of his psychological pathology, however, cannot absolve him of responsibility.

One can only imagine how different the responses to each of these tragedies would have been had Reagan not been as hostile to the gay community, and had Trump not been lost in the grip of his narcissistic personality disorder and enabled by a feckless Republican Senate.

Perhaps the most profound difference between the AIDS and Covid-19 pandemics is in the populations affected. Besides hemophiliacs and IV drug users, the most highly-visible HIV fatalities were gay men. The coronavirus has struck more than such a minority—the world's entire population is at risk and there has been an all-out, multi-national effort to find a cure, treatment and vaccine. With HIV, on the other hand, even as late as the 1990s, there was scattered resistance to HIV study and treatment. AIDS was, after all, the "gay disease." One of my colleagues once gave a lecture on HIV in central Indiana only to have many of the physicians in attendance walk out in a display of disgust and disapproval—the stigma of those infected with HIV was of greater importance than the disease itself. It's difficult to believe that desperate appeals for research and affordable treatment would have been necessary, had the general population been battling AIDS.

Although we may congratulate ourselves on the end of racial discrimination, both the HIV and the Covid-19 epidemics expose the continuing prejudices of our society. It is clear that with the coronavirus, people of color are becoming infected and dying at a rate far greater than white Americans. Nationwide, African-Americans are 13% of our population, but make up over 24% of coronavirus deaths—in places these deaths are more than three times this number. Insurance records show that when Black and white people with Covid-19 symptoms, like fever and coughing, seek medical care, Black people are much less likely to be given a coronavirus test. Researchers think that this isn't due to overt racism, but only the underlying problem of subconscious bias.[9] We know that African-American, Hispanic and Native American people have no inherent genetic susceptibility to either of the two viruses, but rather the differences in their outcomes are due to their general state of baseline poor health and impaired access to medical care.[10] Research indicates that Black people get sick at younger ages, have more severe illnesses and are aging, biologically, more rapidly than whites.[11] People with the lowest incomes have considerably higher rates of diabetes, obesity, asthma, high blood pressure, and kidney and pulmonary disease—and they are caught in patterns of suboptimal care and are much more likely to die from Covid-19, as compared to wealthy Americans.[12]

Why doesn't the US have the same universal healthcare as, literally, every other modern democracy? There is only one reason: race. White Americans principally have not wanted significant resources funneled to the poor, whom they have identified as African-Americans. Investing in safety nets and human capital became stigmatized because of a perception that African-Americans

ANDREW M. FAULK, M.D.

would benefit. Instead of investing in our children, we invested in a personal responsibility narrative holding that Americans just need to lift themselves up by their bootstraps. This was devastating for all Americans, especially the working class. Underinvestment in health and the lack of safety nets means that American children today are 57% more likely to die by age 19 than European children are. America's original sin, slavery, continues to distort and damage the country to this very day.[13]

* * *

We live in a suffocating atmosphere of chronic stress, necessary distance from people and stay-at-home limitations. Covid-19, with its high fatality rate and easy communicability, is a perfect focus for conspiracy theories. In a world turned upside down, conspiracy thinking combats our feelings of confusion and helplessness, giving us a sense of control in a world without control and making us feel safer in a world without safety.

In my practice I'd occasionally encounter someone who saw the world through the lens of conspiracies. Little was known about AIDS for many years and, as both the government and the news were either indifferent or homophobic, rumors came and went. The most common HIV theories involved government biowarfare labs which singled out the gay and African-American communities for destruction or experimentation. Early on, "Chinese Compound Q" was a frequent topic of conversation with a few of my patients, but as I was seen as part of the "establishment," my arguments were doubted as naïve and unreliable. Conspiracy theories foster the belief that the only protection from disease comes from possessing truths that "they" don't want us to hear—that people must find truth on their own. As time passed I heard fewer and fewer rumors, although my gay African-American patients seemed to believe in conspiracy theories longer than did my white patients.

Early in the HIV epidemic, many didn't believe that AIDS was one disease caused by one organism. This was easier to see because of its different manifestations, although the commonality in timing and targets was hard to look past. The belief that the disease was divorced from infection gave cover to continuing incautious behavior. After the causative agent was determined, however, those denying that HIV produced AIDS took on evangelical fervor.

With HIV, conspiracy theories continue to detonate, but such rumblings are like firecrackers when compared to the nuclear bombs of Covid-19. With the coronavirus there are new problems my colleagues and I never had with HIV rumors. Today's Covid-19 conspiracies are turbocharged by the engine of social media. They can originate with any person or government, travel with lightning speed around the world, and generate instant belief and acolytes. In general, rumors are usually first posted online and in books and movies, which are frequently made all the more convincing with high-production values. Conspiracy theories are often started by those with questionable motives, such as anti-vaxxers and those protesting stay-at-home orders, who have political agendas. Here, the truth is at a disadvantage because it is next to impossible to prove a negative; it's difficult to prove that a conspiracy theory is not true.

Unlike the AIDS pandemic, with Covid-19 we must contend with foreign actors maliciously manipulating social media to start and spread conspiracy theories. What Russia learned in the US election of 2016 has become more sophisticated and adopted by China and Iran as well. A top State Department official, Lea Gabrielle, testified in Congress on May 22, 2020, that the Kremlin "seeks to weaken its adversaries by manipulating the information in nefarious ways, by polarizing political conversations, and attempting to destroy the public's faith in good governance, independent media, and democratic principles."[14]

Distorted claims and rumors become elevated from individual sites onto broader areas of social media, where they become more difficult to refute. "Verified" celebrities and fringe "experts" manufacture even more credibility. Like right-wing American TV, these rumors gain validity as they ricochet back and forth in the echo chamber created by broadcasters on "news" networks such as Fox and, indeed, Presidential messaging. Peer-to-peer disinformation is another powerful source of rumor. It is a disturbing phenomenon that when these bits of fantasy are heard repeatedly, they tempt people to consider their validity, even when they know them to be false. Frustratingly, rebutting a conspiracy theory may give it greater credibility and spread, but, on the other hand, lack of push-back only enhances believability. It's exasperating that discussion, either pro or con, only amplifies the message further. The fight for truth is not an easy battle.

There is a streak of anti-scientism in the American mindset that contaminates information about Covid-19: people are less likely to be vaccinated and more likely to seek medical advice from friends and family, instead of physicians and scientists. Trump is a man who is strongly predisposed to believe conspiracy theories—he has created his own and repeated those of others. His messages conflict; he announces that he takes hydroxychloroquine while refusing to wear a mask. Trump advocates the dangerous QAnon theory that violence is the only response to a global cabal of powerful, Satan-worshiping elites who control the world and run a child sex ring. Of course with HIV we've had our own snake oil salesmen, but we more frequently heard President Reagan and his followers proposing religious conversion and abstinence. At one point, he remarked "When it comes to preventing AIDS, don't medicine and morality teach the same lessons?" But to his credit, Reagan never recommended any treatment, dubious or otherwise, in the fight against HIV. Trump, on the other hand, repeatedly attempts to bury his culpability and guarantee his re-election with huckster-style marketing of miracle drugs, musings about household disinfectant injections and conflicting messaging about physical distancing. Although previous instruction was clear and sustained, America has learned that its leader doesn't respect truth—whether in giving it or receiving it.

This misdirection from the top has encouraged the reckless shenanigans of, among others, various ministers who insist on continuing to hold mass church services. Besides the President, our modern-day con artists have often been televangelists. Pastor Jim Bakker required a court injunction to stop him selling colloidal silver, which, in his words, "killed" Covid-19 as well as "every pathogen it has ever been tested on, including SARS and HIV."[15]

Conspiratorial thinking usually bears no relationship to reality, but the most powerful rumors exaggerate and misread important trends, rather than deny them. Although the concept of global integration and transnational governance is visibly disintegrating, the manifest wealth and power of a global overclass together with the rise of digital surveillance has persuaded some conservative Christians and Catholics that a "New World Order" is on the horizon.

Images of totalitarian control, church lockdowns and test-and-trace procedures, with Bill Gates and Anthony Fauci the masterminds, fuel apocalyptic paranoia. Many conservatives demonize mask-wearing as liberal manipulation. In today's America, truth is tribal, reality is unreliable.

I was very fond of my patient George Krivacek, but, unfortunately, he fell into the conspiratorial thinking that the only truly effective treatment for AIDS was one without scientific pedigree—"Compound Q." It seems to be a matter of personality dynamics: if adherents believe one conspiracy, they usually accept many. George was not someone predisposed to entertaining such rumors, but he nonetheless developed a conviction that "Compound Q" was effective. The feelings of security and serenity offered by such rumors may be comforting, but such consolation is fleeting and damage to the public trust is all too real. Such arguments can influence people to take fatal remedies. George Krivacek died pursuing a fantasy cure.

* * *

As the causative agent for AIDS wasn't initially known, people were reluctant to touch someone with the disease or breathe the air in their proximity. By 1984, however, close contact was determined to be safe (except sexual contact), although certain respiratory therapy protocols remained in place after routes of infection were known. A palpable change occurred in 1987 when Princess Diana, ungloved, shook the hand of a man with AIDS. This gesture was a profoundly important step in easing the public's mind.

It is a sad irony of history that at present, Princess Diana's handshake would not signal safety but rather hazard.

The lessons we learned from HIV may not have sunk into society with the depth and reach we may like, but it is well known that sexual intimacy can be dangerous. Covid-19 may be acquired by breathing contaminated air, or possibly touching contaminated surfaces. This extraordinary ease of transmission forces isolation of our sick—exactly when we are in greatest need of physical closeness, we are left to communicate with our loved ones through glass or device.

Between the damage to our bodies and the speed of progression,

ANDREW M. FAULK, M.D.

it's not uncommon for someone to die shortly after being brought to a hospital. Covid-19 teaches us that we cannot refrain from telling our loved ones what they mean to us because we may never see them again. Its speed can rob us of those last moments of time and touch, and frequently those we love step off the earth without the comfort of our presence. The coronavirus is brutal; we cannot hold the hands of our dying.

* * *

When America finally emerges from the medical and economic devastation of Covid-19, we will have an opportunity to build both a more equitable society and a more effective healthcare system. Smaller plagues than this have produced major changes in civilizations. We must always remember, however, that while the world-wide Great Depression of the 1930s gave us Roosevelt's New Deal, it also gave us Hitler's Third Reich.[16]

The Covid-19 crisis has exposed our federal government's lack of resources, competence and ambition. The epidemic has brought many of America's problems into sharp focus and it has exposed the severe inequities of wealth, medical care and policing. Our nation is afflicted by massive, entrenched economic inequality. A great divide separates affluent Americans—who fully enjoy the benefits of life in one of the wealthiest nations on earth—from the growing portion of the population whose lives lack stability or any prospect of betterment. Among western industrialized nations, the United States stands out for the extent of its wealth inequality. At present, the top one percent of our society owns 40% of the nation's wealth. This is twice that of the top one percent in France, Canada or the U.K., and more than three times as much as that of Finland. One American owns six houses around the world, while another sleeps in his car. Is this not societal insanity?

Inequalities of wealth have produced inequalities of health. A middle-aged American in the top fifth of the income distribution can expect to live 13 years longer than a person of the same age in the bottom fifth—a difference that has more than doubled since 1980.[17] The coronavirus has exposed our present healthcare system to be fragile, fragmented and chaotic. Although the United States may spend more than any other industrialized nation on healthcare (and this funding increases at a rate greater than inflation), we have the worst health outcomes and the lowest life expectancy of comparable nations of the west. According to a 2019 report by the World Health Organization, US life expectancy in 2018 was 78.9 years, 38th out of the 186 nations of the world.

We may spend the most, but our spending is not evenly distributed among our citizens. The quality of medical care in the US is based on health insurance, which depends on one's income. Before the pandemic, approximately 10% of Americans did not have insurance. Studies by Harvard's T. H. Chan School of Public Health shows that health insurance is vital for optimum healthcare. Good health insurance can prevent thousands of premature deaths and encourage more than 650,000 Americans to control chronic conditions such as diabetes, high blood pressure and high cholesterol.[18] President Obama's landmark Patient Protection and Affordable Care Act (ACA, Obamacare) clearly decreased health insurance inequalities in the US—particularly for minorities.[19] The ACA has given these newly-insured people access to preventive care, prescription drugs, and doctors' office visits, which has decreased hospital stays and emergency department admissions. In addition, those insured have reported lower rates of depression. By requiring insurance companies to cover people regardless of pre-existing conditions, Obamacare was a huge force in leveling the financial disparity between the sick and the well. Except for those impoverished adults living in states that have rejected ACA Medicaid expansion, e.g. Texas, almost every American can now afford health insurance.

In 2013, before the ACA, 13.3% of Americans were without health insurance; in 2017 thanks to the ACA, the percentage of uninsured fell to 7.9%. But at this moment, the Trump administration is in court suing to end the ACA. For the nine members of the Supreme Court to end the insurance of 23 million Americans, especially during the pandemic, would be particularly cruel. Without Obamacare, many Americans would no longer have insurance because of pre-existing conditions. As more information comes to light, it appears that many of the survivors of the coronavirus may be left with permanent sequelae. These people would lose their insurance precisely because of pre-existing conditions they acquired courtesy of Republican mismanagement of the pandemic.

Although the ACA has done much to provide Americans with

affordable healthcare, often the cost continues to be prohibitive; the majority of bankruptcies in America (66.5%) are due to medical charges. One might imagine that America's healthcare costs are so high because of our extra administration fees and excessive use of CT and MRI scans. These costs are indeed high, but the largest single difference is the cost of medications: we pay more for these than any other developed country in the world.[20]

Pharmaceutical companies blame the high cost of medications on research expenses, but sales of the top 20 drugs pay for all their research plus another 50% over that. Virtually no drug is developed without government subsidization and thus we consumers pay for our medications twice: once from our taxes and once from our wallets. The top 25 pharmaceutical companies report after-expenses profits of 22%, while, in comparison, Amazon's profits are less than five percent.[21] In the US, a one-year supply of insulin costs more than $1,200, yet it's estimated that $130 a year would cover production costs as well as a reasonable profit.[22] Despite such industry profits, many diabetics are forced to ration their insulin. And they are not alone, 24% of adult Americans in fair or poor health must skip or alter their medication dosages because of costs.[23] These human beings are asked to make ultimate sacrifices so that drug companies can afford stock dividends and another yacht for their CEOs. Although virtually all Americans need reductions in drug costs, Congress hasn't protected us from these obscene prices. There are, after all, five pharmaceutical lobbyists for every congressperson.

We don't pay more because of research. We don't pay more because of production costs. *We pay more because pharmaceutical companies charge us more.*

* * *

While the coronavirus puts the entire society at risk, the peril is not spread equally. The social and economic effects of Covid-19 vary markedly by class, and less affluent Americans bear the brunt in health and expense. People of color suffer higher rates of economic fall out than whites. Pew Research Center reports that 61% of low income Hispanic workers say they or someone in their household has lost a job or taken a pay cut; this compares to 44% of low income Black people and 38% of low income whites.[24] At a time when the authorities have advocated staying home as the best way to avoid infection, people of color disproportionately belong to part of the work force that does not have the luxury of working from home. According to the University of Chicago, 37% of jobs in the US can be performed from home, that leaves about two-thirds of workers who must expose themselves to the virus in order to work.

While everyone else is sheltering indoors, these are people who are compelled to serve on the front lines of society—police officers, firefighters, utility maintenance workers, postal workers, janitors, grocery store workers, delivery people and sanitation workers to name a few. They are currently risking their lives because many of them need the income and we need their services. Shamefully, in revoking stay-at-home orders, some states end unemployment benefits for those that refuse to return to work for fear of infection.

Healthcare workers jeopardize their lives as they serve without proper personal protective equipment (PPE), sufficient testing or rest between shifts. In the AIDS epidemic, there was no shortage of medical supplies and our medical workers weren't risking their lives. But at present 12% of hospitalized Covid-19 patients and the dead are medical workers we sent into exam rooms, often with little else than their unshakeable commitment to humanity.[25]

Instead of receiving universal healthcare, hazard pay, decent wages, personal protective equipment, universal paid sick leave and adequate unemployment insurance, our "essential" workers are treated as "expendable" workers. Dr. Martin Luther King, Jr., with astonishing prescience, called for an increase in wages, healthcare, job safety and economic equality when he addressed the striking sanitation workers in Memphis in 1968: "One day our society will come to respect the sanitation worker if it is to survive, for the person who picks up our garbage, in the final analysis, is as significant as the physician, for if he doesn't do his job, diseases are rampant. All labor has dignity."[26]

* * *

Besides highlighting deficiencies in our healthcare system, the coronavirus has also revealed that our democracy is under significant strain. After World War II, there was a greater equality in our incomes and in our society. But during the Reagan presidency, taxes on the most wealthy began to fall from the top tax bracket of 70% in 1979 to 37% at present. These changes have produced differences in wealth that have done much harm to our national community and its politics. This structure helps convince the rich that they've earned their affluence while ignoring their superior educational opportunities as well as stability in health, food and housing. We have all heard some wealthy, and also some impoverished, explain that the rich deserve their wealth because of their hard work. But much of the wealth of the rich is due to financial transactions and income from investments, rather than labor. The more we believe that our success is our own doing, the less likely we are to feel that we owe our fellow citizens. Anyone who has watched a farm worker harvest vegetables knows that this work is backbreaking. Wouldn't it be more fair to tax on the basis of wealth, carbon and financial transactions, instead of wages?

I once asked a cab driver in Copenhagen how much he was taxed. He responded that his 55% would no doubt astonish an American. But he lived a life without anxiety: his medications and his wife's breast cancer treatments were free, one daughter was getting a Ph.D. without school loan burdens, another daughter was receiving child-care and his mother with Alzheimer's received free care. My cab driver lived without debilitating worry. He lived in Denmark, one of the happiest nations on earth, where mutual obligation, what each citizen owes each other, is revered. He asked me, pointedly, how much money did he need?

Besides an inequality of taxes, much of the difference in wealth is based on differences in level of education. The deepest and most persistent divide in our nation is income inequality and some researchers insist that it's not only lack of education that produces poverty, but it's the attendant lack of opportunity.[27] These two go hand in hand. Without education, opportunities are out of reach and one is limited to low-wage jobs, substandard housing and poor diets. People of color make up the largest proportion of the poor, because basic education is often outside their reach. In our country, with all its wealth, many Americans need to work two or three jobs to support a family. In recent decades, governing elites have done little to ensure that the poor are paid a living wage nor granted them the respect they deserve.

The epidemic has highlighted how our political class,

disproportionately white and wealthy, is protected from disease and poverty. In 2018 the median wealth of a US senator was $3.2 million and $900,000 for a member of the House of Representatives.[28] In uncanny divination, in February, 2016, Peggy Noonan wrote in *The Wall Street Journal*, "The protected make public policy, the unprotected live in it." Tragically, as money is the foundation of our political system, the wealthy and corporations control our taxes, economics, medical care and, of course, our political system itself.

In dominating our politics, the rich write preferential legislation which not only favors them, but in so doing undermines the rule of law. Our Congress responds to wealthy donors more than public opinion. With entrenched corruption and indifference, the Senate debated for weeks before finally coming up with a "rescue" bill that gave billions to corporations and banks, while giving the poor and middle class funds that would perhaps pay rent for one or two months, but little more. These officials voted one-time stimulus checks of around $1,200 and for augmented unemployment to expire at the end of July, 2020, as if that were enough to sustain workers, whose median income is $61,973.

It is a universal understanding in America that the rich live under different rules than the poor—the average American, correctly, takes it for granted that in our system of justice, it is better to have money than innocence. Especially under Trump and Attorney General William Barr, one can betray the entire country and face a sentence of a mere four months or less, while a car accident or cannabis possession can result, under certain circumstances, in 22 years. Millions of people lost their homes in the devastating financial crisis of 2008, yet not one person responsible spent one night in jail. Meanwhile the banks and financial houses, led by Goldman Sachs, were able to reward their directors with bonuses the size of many countries' GDP.

Inequalities of class, money and power have produced resentment in those without these advantages. We live in a dangerously polarized country that has become more so as financial and judicial inequality has increased. People no longer belong to political parties based on policy differences, now they are chosen based according to "tribe." Trump's populist clan disdains educational and financial elites who have abused the rule of law and the disadvantaged. Our political system must address these divisions, or the underlying forces that

270

produced the wreckage of our present politics will remain and we will have more Trumps. And future Trumps may be much more dangerous to democracy—more intelligent, strategic and self-disciplined."

* * *

Nicola (Chris) Bucci, our friend in San Quentin, remains imprisoned there. In April, 2020, California's worst coronavirus pandemic occurred at the men's prison in Chino, east of Los Angeles. In attempting to quell this outbreak, hundreds of inmates were transferred to San Quentin, but the transfer was done without adequate testing of those being transferred and now it is San Quentin that is suffering the State's worst Covid-19 outbreak. In fact, it is the nation's third largest outbreak. Since the first cases of the coronavirus were reported at the end of June, more than one-third of the inmates and staff—1,600 people—have tested positive. Twelve have died.

San Quentin, like most prisons in the nation, is overcrowded, with inmates living in dormitory settings with shared bathrooms, showers and telephones. The cells are cramped and almost none of the cells have walls on all sides; nearly all the men must breathe the same ventilated air. For safety, cleaning supplies can't contain alcohol or bleach, making basic sanitation harder.

Governor Gavin Newsom has ordered the release of 8,000 prisoners who are at high risk of complications or scheduled to be released soon. But motions in federal courts to compel Newsom to release these prisoners have been denied and his order has been carried out at a glacial pace. Jay Jordan, executive director of Californians for Safety and Justice, has said, "It's ironic that California has a moratorium on the death penalty, yet people are being killed in prisons by way of COVID." Many are older men living in cramped spaces and breathing the same ventilated air. With the coronavirus advancing through their ranks, they are falling one after the next. One inmate who was released in early July had this to say: "When I left, I saw grown men crying. They were thinking they weren't going to see their grandkids anymore. Like I didn't get the death penalty. I'm scared…"

Bucci tested positive for Covid-19 in late June and since then he has been quarantined in a cell usually set aside for those in solitary confinement.

The situation is dire. Bucci never complains, but in one of the rare phone calls he was allowed before they took away the right to make calls, he reluctantly admitted that the conditions are "even worse than just being held in solitary." Food vendors have now refused to come to the prison, so food supplies are low; many of the kitchen staff have become infected and are no longer working. Correctional officers are working double and even triple shifts. Doctors have been working 12-plus-hour days, seven days a week, for the past six weeks. Public Defender Mary McComb writes, "Men (including some who have tested positive) report not having access to doctors, not receiving medication for symptoms such as coughs, and not receiving regular oxygen-level or blood pressure checks. San Quentin's staff—especially medical staff—is simply drowning among the chaos."

Bucci gets three bagged meals a day, if you can call them meals. For breakfast he gets six crackers and a small stick of cheese. For lunch and dinner the menu is two slices of bread, two slices of bologna, two cheese-type crackers and two chocolate chip cookies. The cell blocks are always noisy and loud as inmates are hungry, angry and yelling for food and services.

Bucci has a parole hearing mid-July when we fully expect he'll be found suitable for parole—he has been a model prisoner, he is no danger to society, and he has paid dearly for causing a car accident 13 ½ years ago that didn't involve drugs or alcohol. Frank and I have notified the Parole Board that we will provide him a place to live and employment. Even if parole is granted, inmates are normally retained another four months. We don't know if that time will be shortened for him or not.

Bucci remains one of the most positive and optimistic men I know. Incarceration can drain the life out of a man. For Bucci it has not. He is a remarkable man: his patience, optimism and happiness, in light of his surroundings, are astonishing.

Prison authorities say San Quentin's ongoing crisis should offer stark warnings for prisons and jails across the nation, many of which are now struggling to handle their own outbreaks. As our nation imprisons more people, per capita, than any other nation on earth, it is imperative to reform our criminal justice system.

* * *

ANDREW M. FAULK, M.D.

When it comes to developing a fairer political world, medical care is a good place to start. A first step to reform is to change the way we think about the healthcare system. Healthcare isn't determined by routine free market mechanisms: a test, hospital or doctor isn't truly chosen. For the average person, insurance plans and deductibles limit choices of physician and medication. Increasingly, large healthcare corporations are monopolies which control doctor and hospital fees. Free-market capitalism is based on individuals freely choosing products, but the only true choices we have when it comes to medical care is which insurance policy to select. People of the right may argue that government involvement interferes with the efficiency of free-market capitalism, but in fact it is uncontrolled capitalism that has given us the highest costs and worst care of any industrialized nation.

Our citizens are convinced of the superior benefit of insurance through their employer as if insurance were a gift. In actuality, this system robs them of the higher wages they've earned and transfers it to pharmaceutical companies and for-profit medical conglomerates. It would be more accurate to think of employer-provided health insurance as a tax. The American healthcare system has not been good at promoting health, but it has excelled at taking money from all of us for its benefit. Companies have one defining motivation—they exist to make profit. *Shouldn't our medical system be motivated to provide the best healthcare for us, rather than the most profit for a corporation?*

After this era of pandemic sorrow and leadership failure, we may be able to obtain what our unresponsive government has long blocked—acknowledgement of medical care as a human right.

In our coronavirus calamity the free market has failed to protect us, but so have our disengaged political leaders. The US had warnings from epidemiologists and examples from Europe which could have offered us a chance at mitigation or even containment rather than this suicidal course to herd immunity. Government coordination and planning would have allowed our hospitals to prepare with PPE and ventilators, laboratories to be ready with functioning tests, and structures in place for contact tracing and quarantines. Trump has always placed his own interests ahead of those of the nation, and he made the flawed and faithless choice to protect the stock market rather than our people. But he has had a political advantage for many months: when people are in a crisis and deeply worried, support for leaders increases and individuals seek solace in national unity. We are motivated to see the world as a secure and stable place, and anxiety can be soothed by joining a strong group with the appearance of a strong leader.

But Trump wasn't alone in culpability: our Republican Senate failed the people of America. When Trump was impeached, there was no true dispute that he was extraordinarily unfit to be president. The Senate refused to hear even one witness. It was on Feb. 5, 2020, that 53 Republican Senators acquitted him and allowed him to remain in office.

* * *

Trump's malignant nonsense has exposed what we desperately need from leadership: example, honesty, empathy and vision. When a president lies and asks more of us than he does of himself, our faith in institutions is damaged—we become cynical and our commitment to a common goal is harmed. Leading by example defends us against feelings of inequality and shows us our shared responsibilities to each other. When a leader strives to quell differences, the best comes out in us. Honesty and clarity defend us against being overwhelmed by obstacles and limitations; they block premature surrender. Vision inspires us to see beyond ourselves and our present difficulties. When weaknesses and despair are acknowledged, we see the humanity and nobility in our leaders. When a president admits ignorance, we respond to his humility and honesty with greater faith in his pronouncements. Truth and transparency deflate corrosive conspiracy theories. When a president leads us in collective mourning, we acknowledge our fundamental interdependency and shared ethical responsibility for the physical lives of each other. When we allow ourselves to recognize the full significance of those we've lost, we build a foundation for solidarity and collective action. With great leadership we celebrate our kinship and recognize our shared responsibility for each other; we endure sacrifice for a common goal.

Military expenditures have not purchased our safety: Covid-19 has slaughtered more of our countrymen than many of our wars combined and left us to suffer an economic depression the likes of

ANDREW M. FAULK, M.D.

which hasn't been seen since the 1930s. The CDC, which may have saved us, was starved into incompetence and irrelevance by our politicians, while each year Congress votes for an armed forces budget wildly out of step with the nation's needs. US financial planning for 2020 reveals that our country will spend more on our military than that of the next 10 countries combined—a questionable investment when our military establishment has proven that, without question or hesitancy, it will turn its resources against the American people.[29]

White people have been victimized by our militarized police only of late, but Black people have suffered from its duplicity, arrogance and power for generations. We are seeing a tremendous shift in society with the Black Lives Matter movement, the largest movement in American history, which has approximately 20 million adherents. The picture of a man being killed by another one planting a knee on his neck is a powerful image. Even white people have become disgusted by the casual murder of Black people by police forces which appear to operate without accountability. There is evidence that Black Lives Matter and the catastrophes of Trump and the coronavirus are making a difference in the political climate of the US. A CBS News poll in June, 2020, showed 60% of Americans, including a majority of white Americans, support ideas of the Black Lives Matter movement. A 56% majority supports a national healthcare plan, and 89% favor higher taxes on the wealthy to reduce poverty in America.[30]

Perhaps the medical and economic disaster of the coronavirus may finally awaken Americans as to how their money is being spent. It could be that our society will re-evaluate our wars abroad and rethink our involvement and goals. Surely the national budget requires a second look when the cost of one more aircraft carrier can fund all of the nation's "Head Start" programs (pre-kindergarten food and services) for an entire year? Money could be directed away from the endless production of fighter jets, many so poorly designed that they can't fly, and towards funding national healthcare, child care, psychiatric services and care for the elderly.

It could be that, instead of American flag decals plastered on the back windows of our SUVs, we genuinely support our troops by ending our wars and bringing our service members home. Surely we've learned by now that wars produce humanitarian disasters and hatred of our nation, and that their horrendous brutality and violence leave our soldiers physical and emotional wrecks. Furthermore these unconstitutional, casual wars create in our people a poisonous intoxication of power that degrades our sense of the value of human life. Haven't we learned that it is out of condescension and ignorance that we "teach" other nations democracy with bombs and bullets?

Do the American people really want "Made In America" to be stenciled on the shrapnel found among the hundreds of people slaughtered at a wedding half-way round the world?

The American sense of exceptionalism cannot remain the same. Either it will remain mass delusion and we will accept the Trump lie that the American response to Covid-19 has been "great," or we will recognize that our country is exceptional only in the sense of our willingness to accept a profoundly unfair and undemocratic system—a system which has cursed us with some of the worst leadership in the western world and a medical system hopelessly inadequate to face the tragedy of the coronavirus or any other future pandemic.

* * *

We are made spiritually and emotionally richer when we give of ourselves and our resources to those physically and financially troubled. In one of the richest nations on earth, must we consign our less fortunate neighbors to depend on an income which is undependable? Shouldn't we apply Christ's admonition to "love your neighbor as you love yourself" to the impoverished and mentally ill, who live outside on our streets and underneath our freeway on-ramps. Perhaps in the future there may be no need for "GoFundMe" pages to raise money for overwhelming hospital bills. It's possible that there will no longer be need for donations to food banks for those without work or bank accounts. It may be that there won't be bins in grocery store parking lots for food, clothing and children's Christmas toys. There is a reason we use the term "less fortunate"— we know that the majority of these people have had skirmishes with bad luck. It could be that, in a refreshed America, we prove our protestations of love and brotherhood are more than meaningless, formulaic expressions and demonstrate these values as we fill out our ballots.

Our struggle with HIV is helping prepare us for what is to

ANDREW M. FAULK, M.D.

come. With AIDS, society built an American order in which gay people have a crucial role. Importantly, the HIV pandemic led to the mainstreaming of condom use and STD testing and it underscored the drawbacks of casual intimacy. The disclosures of the HIV pandemic led to stunning advances in gay acceptance and legal acknowledgement of our community. As a product of a different social and political time, I find myself amazed that I am legally married to my husband and can refer to him using that word and announce our relationship without encountering hostility or sarcasm. Whether it be a waiter or a tennis star, the mailman or the neighbor, the president or the other driver in a fender bender, I speak my truth without experiencing a fragment of antagonism or confrontation; my orientation is neither an issue of significance nor disparagement. No one can tell me to leave my spouse's hospital room because I am not a relative. While acceptance of gay people did not occur worldwide, it did find a home in the US and in the industrialized nations of the west. ACT UP's demands helped bring about changes in the way we provide for those with AIDS, in what scientists do research on, and how we think about LGBTQ rights; it left its mark on peaceful protest, successful activism and pride in the defense of our brothers and sisters and our community. ACT UP gave our entire society "compassionate use" drug approval in those cases of near hopelessness. Without ACT UP's demands on behalf of AIDS patients, the legalization of cannabis would no doubt have been delayed until white America awoke to the immorality of mass incarceration of Black people, resulting from the nefarious "War on Drugs."

As we have learned from the pandemic of HIV, periods of social upheaval carry with them great potential. Hopefully the pandemic will be a force in recognizing the worth of all individuals, especially people of color, the elderly, the sick, the disabled and the imprisoned. Our struggle with the economic devastation of Covid-19 may become a powerful force in creating an economy that honors the dignity of work by paying salaries high enough to raise families and protect us from sudden misfortune.

It is possible we may create a society where *all* our people are recognized as essential workers.

* * *

If the HIV pandemic has taught us anything, it is that our health and safety depend on collective action. Dr. Anthony Fauci has said "If we don't extinguish the outbreak, sooner or later, even [states] that are doing well are going to be vulnerable to the spread, the only way we're going to end [the pandemic] is by ending it together."[31] It is possible that the America we build will be based on the humanity of shared hope and vulnerability, the humility of the precariousness of life, and the courage and resilience of fighting a foreign occupier on our soil. The coronavirus pandemic will almost certainly result in more extensive societal changes than those that accompanied AIDS.

In state capitals, armed right-wing demonstrators protest stay-at-home orders and face-mask ordinances as "assaults on freedom." It is clear they have a minimalist concept of what liberty means—a photo-negative view of freedom. Their definition means a freedom from civic duty, freedom from mutual obligation, freedom from caring for our sick, elderly and poor. This is a definition of the word which has been used to protect wealth and privilege.

As pandemics engulf us with terrible repercussions, there is hope.

Covid-19's devastating onslaught spurs us to create a society based on common freedoms: freedom of racial equality, socio-economic justice, and universal access to medical care.

In the past other invisible micro-organisms have attacked us with as much deadly force as a visible military invasion. We have faced much hardship, and are destined to face more with future pandemics. We will all achieve a greater understanding of this horror: this pandemic. Our pandemic. But from this point in history, we'll also achieve a fuller, more complete understanding of the word "freedom." An understanding that none of us are free unless all of us are free, that none of us are safe unless all of us are safe. That we are, truly, all in this together.

ANDREW M. FAULK, M.D.

ENDNOTES

[1] Since its discovery in 1981, AIDS has become one of the world's greatest public health concerns. Human immunodeficiency virus (HIV) targets CD4+ T-cells, causing a steady decline in the absolute number of these cells with progressive immune deficiency as a result. The T-cell count (CD4 count) is the laboratory test generally accepted as the best indicator of the immediate state of immunologic competence of those with HIV infection. I have used lone numbers for T-cell counts (e.g., "200") when, in actuality, I mean the number of CD4 T-cells per cubic mm. A normal CD4 T-cell count is 500/cubic mm to 1,200/cubic mm.

Another important marker of possible disease progression is "viral burden," or "viral load," which is the quantity of virus particles identified in a patient's blood. The more HIV there is in blood, then the faster the CD4 cell count will fall, and the greater one's risk of becoming ill because of HIV.

[2] American Centers for Disease Control (CDC) statistics. From 1981 through 1992, AIDS caused approx. 229,000 American deaths. From 1981 through 2000, there were approx. 448,000 deaths in the US. Worldwide, as of 2020, there have been 32 million deaths from HIV and it is estimated that 37 million people live with the infection.

[3] One method for interrupting obsessive thinking, advised by Dr. Kathryn Korslund, an expert in Dialectical Behavior Therapy, is to dip one's face in ice water. This activates the parasympathetic nervous system which lowers body temperature and heart rate and interrupts emotions from intensifying.

[4] "Crix Belly"—The particular lipodystrophy phenomenon of the accumulation of fat in the abdomen named after the medication Crixivan which was thought to be the primary cause. It's now well established that other antiretrovirals, alone or in combination, can create the same condition.

[5] Frankl, Viktor, *Man's Search for Meaning*. Boston, Beacon Press, 1959 and 2006. Pp. 120-121.

[6] Ibid., pg. 83.

[7] Willoughby, Teena. "Examining the Link Between Adolescent Brain Development and Risk Taking From a Social-Developmental Perspective." *Brain Cogn*, 89:70-8, (Aug., 2014).

[8] Johnson, Steven. "Report: Public Health Funding Falls Despite Increasing Threats." *Modern Healthcare*, (4/24/19);

Wahowiak, Lindsey. "President's proposed budget disastrous for public health: Prevention, ACA progress threatened." *The Nation's Health*, 48 (2): 1-16, (April 2018).

[9] Farmer, Blake. "The Coronavirus Doesn't Discriminate, But U.S. Health Care Showing Familiar Biases." *Health News from NPR*, (April 2, 2020).

[10] Lavizzo-Mourey, Risa and David Williams. "Being Black is Bad for Your Health." *U.S. News & World Report*, (4/14/2016).

[11] Ibid.

[12] "Preliminary Estimates of the Prevalence of Selected Underlying Health Conditions Among Patients with Coronavirus Disease 2019—United States, February 12–March 28, 2020." *MMWR Morb Mortal Wkly Rep* 2020;69:382–386, (February 12–March 28, 2020).

[13] Thakrar, Ashish and Alexandra Forrest. "Child Mortality in the US and 19 OECD Comparator Nations: A 50-year Time-Trend Analysis." *Health Affairs*. Vol. 37, No. 1 (January, 2018)

[14] Romm, Tony. "State Dept. Blames Swarms of Online False Personas' from Russia for Wave of Commission for Information Online." *The Washington Post*, (March 5, 2020).

[15] Colloidal silver causes argyria, a permanent bluish-gray discoloration of the skin. It also interacts dangerously with hydroxychloroquine.

[16] The United States is well on its way to fascism. As I write this, before the election of 2020, American democracy is threatened by a powerful combination of forces aligned against it: President Donald Trump, Attorney General William Barr, the Republican Party, conservative right-wing media such as Fox News and the governments of China and Russia. But even should the President and the Republican Party be defeated in the election, the underlying forces that produced the wreckage of our present politics will remain: legitimate differences in policy will persist as all-consuming issues of tribe and virtue. When honest information is demonized as propaganda and unbiased news is discredited as "the enemy of the people," when objective facts and demonstrable science are

ANDREW M. FAULK, M.D.

disparaged as elitism, productive discourse and peaceful comity become nearly impossible.

[17] Ichiro Kawachi, John L. Loeb and Frances Lehman Loeb Professor of Social Epidemiology, Harvard's T.H. Chan School of Public Health, Department of Social and Behavioral Sciences. "The costs of inequality: Money = quality health care = longer life." *The Harvard Gazette*, (Feb. 22, 2016).

[18] McDonough, John and Thomas McGuire. Harvard's T. H. Chan School of Public Health. "The costs of inequality: Money = quality health care = longer life." *The Harvard Gazette*, (Feb. 22, 2016).

[19] Ibid.

[20] Danzon, Patricia and Sean Nicholson. *The Economics of the Biopharmaceutical Industry*. London: Oxford University Press and Liverpool University, 2012.

[21] Adams, Christopher and Van Brantner. "Estimating the Cost of new drug development: is it really $802 million?" *Health Affairs*. Vol. 25, no. 2, (March/April 2006).

[22] Danzon, Patricia and Sean Nicholson, *The Economics of the Biopharmaceutical Industry*. London, Oxford University Press and Liverpool University, 2012.

[23] Henry J. Kaiser Family Foundation. *National Health Issues*, (March 1, 2019).

[24] Parker, Kim and Juliana Horowitz. "Household Job or Wage Loss to COVID-19." *Social and Demographic Changes*, Pew Research Center, (April 21, 2020).

[25] Stone, Will and Carrie Feibel. "COVID-19 Has Killed Close To 300 U.S. Health Care Workers, New Data From CDC Shows." *Health News from NPR*, (May 28, 2020).

[26] King, M. L., Jr. Presentation at the Second National Convention of the Medical Committee for Human Rights, Chicago, (3/25/1966).

[27] Ichiro Kawachi, John L. Loeb and Frances Lehman Loeb Professor of Social Epidemiology, Harvard's T.H. Chan School of Public Health, Department of Social and Behavioral Sciences. "The costs of inequality: Money = quality health care = longer life." *The Harvard Gazette*, (Feb. 22, 2016).

[28] Kopf, Dan. "The typical US Congress member is 12 times richer than the typical American household." *Quartz Daily Brief*, (Feb. 12, 2018).

[29] On June 1, 2020, US Attorney General William Barr, under the direction of President Donald Trump, deployed the D.C. National Guard, Secret Service and notorious Park Police against peaceful protesters in

Washington, D.C. These troops, in riot gear, were ordered into the streets armed with, among other things, firearms with bayonets. Days later, Gen. Mark Milley, chairman of the Joint Chiefs of Staff, and Defense Secretary, Mark Esper, released a "strongly worded statement" against this mobilization. There were other troops which wore no insignia and would not say which branch of the government or military they represented. Secret police were also used against the general populace in mid-July, 2020, in Portland, Oregon.

[30] Backus, Fred and Jennifer De Pinto, Anthony Salvanto, Kabir Khanna, Elena Cox. "Majority Agree with Black Lives Matter and say major police reform is needed—CBS News poll." *CBS News*, (June 28, 2020);

"Public Opinion on Single-Payer, National Health Plans, and Expanding Access to Medicare Coverage." *KFF (Kaiser Family Foundation)*, (May 27, 2020).

[31] Shear, Michael D. and Maggie Haberman. "New Numbers Showing Coronavirus Spread Intrude on a White House Denial." *The New York Times*, (June 26, 2020).

ANDREW M. FAULK, M.D.

Donations to support AIDS research may be sent to the University of Washington.

ANDREW M. FAULK, M.D.
ENDOWED FUND FOR HIV/AIDS

UNIVERSITY OF WASHINGTON SCHOOL OF MEDICINE

Gifts can be made to the Andrew M. Faulk, M.D. Endowed Fund for HIV/AIDS by searching for that fund on this page:

https://www.washington.edu/giving/make-a-gift

Gifts by check may be made out to "Andrew M. Faulk, M.D. Endowed Fund" and sent to:

UW Medicine Advancement
Attn: Gift Processing
Box 358045
Seattle, WA 98195-8045